A FOOD

REVOLUTION

How the Plant-Based Lifestyle
Can Win the Global War on
Diabetes, Obesity, and Heart Disease

Anita Lesko, BSN, RN, MS, CRNA

Copyright © 2020 by Anita Lesko, BSN, RN, MS, CRNA
Your Whole Food Plant-Based Life: www.yourwfpblife.com
Facebook: The Plant-Based Diva
Instagram: The Plant-Based Diva
Twitter: @anitalesko1
anitalesko1@gmail.com
www.yourwfpblife.com

Printed in the United States of America
Library of Congress Cataloging-in-Publication Data
is available from the publisher, the author Anita Lesko.

ISBN 978-1-7346985-4-1

Disclaimer

This book is intended to be a guide for consideration of an alteration or assumption of a diet that has provided for the author and many others for their best health ever. It is not intended or implied to be a substitute for professional advice, diagnosis, or treatment, or a substitute for healthcare that has been prescribed by your own doctor. Work with your physician or qualified healthcare provider before adjusting medications or making major diet changes. Before any new diet or exercise regime, seek advice from your doctor.

Dedication

I dedicate this book to my mom, Rita, for planting the seeds of the plant-based diet in my mind all those years ago. I only wish I would have listened then. She would probably still be here.

Other Books by Anita Lesko

Asperger's Syndrome: When Life Hands You Lemons, Make Lemonade
iUniverse, 2011

The Complete Guide to Autism & Healthcare
Future Horizons, 2017

Recipient of the Autism Society of America's highest literary award -- the **Temple Grandin Literary Award -** *- The Complete Guide to Autism & Healthcare* is geared to the medical community and other healthcare providers. The book was adopted into the healthcare curriculum coursework by multiple universities/medical schools in an innovative program *in 2018* focusing on the development and insight into the subject of autism for doctors and providers. Data showed a dearth of information on the subject of autism in medical training, which was substantially and negatively impacting the medical care and healthcare programs for those on the autism spectrum.

The Complete Guide to Autism & Healthcare also serves as a guide for healthcare providers who work with those involved in the **Special Olympics** as well as those in law enforcement communities.

Temple Grandin: The Stories I Tell My Friends
Future Horizons 2018.

Becoming an Autism Success Story
Future Horizons 2019

Foreword by Dr. Tony Attwood and A Special Note by Dr. Temple Grandin

Table of Contents

Foreword

By Neal D. Barnard, MD

The world of diabetes has been incontrovertibly changed. Not so many years ago, the disease was considered a one-way street. Once you had diabetes, you would always have diabetes, doctors said. With an ever-increasing armamentarium of medications, they tried only to slow the onslaught of complications: visual problems, neuropathy, and kidney disease. As medication doses climbed higher, patients became discouraged, and their family members worried that genetic tendencies would dictate the same fate for them.

From this dismal scenario has emerged a completely new vista. Research has shown that, in fact, the disease is a two-way street. Blood sugars that have gone up can come back down. The need for medication can diminish, sometimes to the point where no medications are needed at all, and, for all intents and purposes, the disease has gone away.

Where did this answer come from? Not from a new pill, a new kind of insulin, or some new glucose monitoring system. The answer came from rethinking food. In 2003. The National Institutes of Health funded our research team to try to find a better approach to Type 2 Diabetes. Drawing on prior studies that had found that people who generally favored plant-based diets were at much less risk of developing the disease, in contrast to people on meatier diets, who were particularly high risk, we developed new theories about how foods might be able to alter the disease process itself. Our research participants eagerly joined our research studies, hoping to gain more control over their condition. In the course of our research, their lives changed dramatically, and, in the years that followed, it has become commonplace for people to be able to greatly reduce the medications and, sometimes, eliminate them entirely and even see the disappearance of the disease.

In the process, we have come to understand what is happening in the body. Normally, insulin travels from the pancreas through the bloodstream to the cells of the body, where it acts like a key, opening the cell membrane to the entrance of glucose—the simple sugar that acts as a fuel for the cell. As long as insulin is doing its job, it is able to open the cell membrane, and glucose floods from the bloodstream in the cell. However, if fatty foods pack fat particles into the cells, the insulin "key" no longer works. It is as if the lock is jammed—jammed with fat that came from our mealtime choices. With a diet tune-up, all of this can change. The fat that had built up inside the cell can begin to disappear, as does the disease itself.

A technique called "magnetic resonance spectroscopy" allows us to measure the fat inside the cells. As patients put the power of a healthier diet to work, we can watch that fat gradually dissipate and can see patients improve day by day.

This book tells you the experience of someone who has put this new science to work. Like many people, Anita had tried hard with all manner of diets, with increasing frustration. But she learned—as you will, too—that there is a much more effective approach. Anita not only shows you how it worked for her; she shares a step-by-step pathway for putting it to work in your own life.

This book is an immensely practical guide for anyone who would like to put the power of nutrition to work and to regain good health. As a physician, I believe that you will find this information to be lifechanging. And I would ask that you take what you learn here and share it with others who are struggling. You will change their lives, too.

Neal D. Barnard, MD
Adjunct Professor, George Washington University School of Medicine
President, Physicians Committee for Responsible Medicine
202-527-7303

Introduction

Time is of the essence.

There are over 422 million people around the world with Type 2 Diabetes. Diabetes is the 7th leading cause of death in America, affecting 1 in every 3 people. I made the decision to publish this book myself, because every second counts. There's too much at stake: *your life.*

High blood sugar, the result of Type 2 Diabetes, wreaks havoc inside every organ of your body as well as your entire vascular system. It can lead to a host of issues, including heart disease, strokes, heart attacks, kidney failure, blindness, nerve damage, weakened immune system, and amputations. It is not uncommon to be pre-diabetic or even have full-blown diabetes and not recognize it despite many symptoms.

My journey began when I discovered I had Type 2 Diabetes. I was instructed to take diabetes pills to help keep my blood glucose levels under control, Regular insulin, eat a diet that needed to be extremely low in carbohydrates, focus on mostly meat, and zero sugar. Once you're diagnosed with diabetes, these "protocols" of insulin and diet based on meat and protein are the mantra doctors have been using for years to slow down the disease. The Primary Care Physician I was going to at the time told me diabetes was worse than cancer, because "at least many cancers have a cure. Diabetes has none." As a medical professional myself for over 35 years, I always thought of diabetes as a progressive disease "in which there was no cure."

However, there is a successful way to address this disease.

What if I told you that Type 2 Diabetes can be *reversed, WITHOUT DRUGS?* Like most people, you might think, that's impossible. I'm here to tell you, it's not impossible. How do I know? Because I have reversed my diabetes, and there are thousands of others who are doing exactly the same thing.

My journey brought me to a modern-day hero who has helped many diabetics, but, instead of a cape, he wears a white lab coat. Through all his extensive research into Type 2 Diabetes, (with much of it funded by the National Institutes for Health [NIH]), he discovered the true causes of Type 2 Diabetes and how to reverse it without drugs. Dr. Neal Barnard literally saved my life, because I was unable to take any diabetes medications, so my blood sugars were very poorly controlled. I was eating what my doctor had instructed, a Keto-type diet (based on a significant component of meat), and I exercised daily for 30 minutes. Unfortunately, all of this didn't much help.

On my own, I tried but was not successful in searching for a natural way to cure or improve my Type 2 Diabetes. I was also fired by my Primary Care Physician for being "non-compliant," because I wouldn't take all the medications he was prescribing. I literally begged him for an alternative way to control it. He would always repeat himself, stating that diabetes is a progressive disease for which there is no cure. I was feeling sicker with each passing day. I was convinced I was soon going to die, because every step was a major ordeal. I would wake up each morning, feeling like lead was traveling through my veins: nauseated, exhausted, and short of breath. I was in a lot of pain and my future looked grim!

Then everything changed.
Two months after getting fired from my Primary Care Physician, I was introduced to someone who told me about the whole food plant-based diet (WFPBD). She also told me about Dr. Neal Barnard's program of how to reverse Type 2 Diabetes without drugs.

A light bulb went off in my head! Many years earlier, back around 2006, my mom had heard of Dr. Barnard and got his book about diabetes. At that time, I was not ready to listen to her, so I basically tuned out whenever she talked about him and his books. I thought it was just another fad diet. But she planted the seed in my mind, which now suddenly sprung to life! My prayers were answered.

After nearly two years of desperately searching for a natural cure, I realized this was *exactly* what I'd been hoping to find.

I immediately jumped into the whole food plant-based lifestyle. I didn't view it as a diet; it was, simply, a solution! No measuring, no counting calories, no tiny portions, but, most importantly, a definite change of lifestyle. You eat what you want from an extensive list of foods, which create delicious meals. Even more, not only will your blood sugar levels begin to drop, you will start losing weight as well!

In my life, I have tried every diet that has ever been created, yet none of them ever worked for me.

What exactly is the whole food plant-based diet?

It is a diet that consists of whole grains, legumes, vegetables, and fruits. It excludes all animal products: no meat, chicken, pork, fish, and dairy products, such as milk, butter, yogurt, cheese, and eggs. No oils either.

OK. I know exactly what you are thinking. I bet you are envisioning dinners at your favorite steak house, your scrambled eggs and bacon for breakfast, sautéing onions in a slather of butter and more.

You might think life would not be the same without all of those types of food, and you are exactly right: l**ife will be 100%** *better* without it all. It will change your life, give you back energy and your health and, you will experience effortless weight loss if you are overweight.

Best of all, life will be possible without diabetes! This new lifestyle will be the best life insurance policy you could ever have.

This book is not only for those who are patients with Type 2 Diabetes, but physicians and nurses as well. The healthcare providers need to know that **diabetes can be reversed without drugs**. I want to save people from being a victim twice – first, from Type 2 Diabetes and, second, from physicians who lack the knowledge of the power of the whole food plant-based diet. Traditionally, medical students get little if any training about nutrition during their education. While this is changing slowly, it is a long way from being mainstream. Hundreds of millions of people with Type 2 Diabetes need to know their alternatives to this killer disease.

This book will show anyone with Type 2 Diabetes how to adopt the whole food plant-based lifestyle to take control of their health. Healthcare providers have a major impact on this disease, as my near-death experience illustrates as a good example of why physicians need to be educated on the benefits of a whole food plant-based diet. I will share
many ways they can offer alternative treatment methods to their patients, based on Dr. Neal Barnard's model used at the Barnard Medical Center.

The World Health Organization states "There is a globally agreed target to halt the rise in diabetes and obesity by 2025." [1] My dream is to help achieve this goal, which is the purpose of this book.

Knowledge and information will win the global war on diabetes.

Let the battle begin!

Anita Lesko, BSN, RN, MS, CRNA

Part 1 – My Journey to the Plant-Based Lifestyle

Chapter 1 - Last Cheeseburger and Fries

Little did I know my entire life was about to change in the next hour, when I was sitting in my truck in the drive-up at McDonald's to order my lunch. Looking over the menu board, I pretty much already knew what I wanted. Just looking at all the pretty photos of their food was whetting my appetite. Pulling up to order, the human voice happily asked what I'd like.

Looking at the photos of the food as I spoke, "I'd like the Double Quarter Pounder with cheese, extra onions on it, and small fries. And a diet Coke, large."

My intention was not to eat the bun, so I'd cut out carbohydrates to follow my doctor's order; I intended to eat just the meat and cheese along with the fixings. After all, it's the protein that I was told to be eating "to help my diabetes." That concept was, also, the same thing I found in all my endless research for a cure for Type 2 Diabetes. Well, they didn't say to eat cheeseburgers, but they did say to eat lots of protein, eliminate sugars, and only eat less than 50 grams of carbohydrates ("carbs") a day.

I paid at the first window, then pulled forward. It was the height of lunch time, so there were several vehicles ahead of me. As I patiently waited, my thoughts wandered to how America relies on fast food to get them through their day. I knew full well that it isn't healthy to eat fast food, but, in a pinch, it would have to do. Protein and lots of it was my goal for most meals, per doctor's orders. That's what I aimed for throughout my day. That's what I had been taught all my life. We need large amounts of protein to survive, all of which comes from animals.

As I eased up to the window, a smiling young man confirmed my order, then reached out with the brown bag containing my double quarter pounder with cheese, the small fries, and a large diet Coke. I also asked for some salt packets to sprinkle on my fries and burger. At this moment I thought of a co-worker I used to know when I lived in Madison, Wisconsin. Tom treated himself to several supersize cheeseburgers and fries when he'd be on-call for the overnight shift. He would sit down at the table, open the fancy silver wrappers on the burgers, and proceed to shake on enough salt to make it look like Jack Frost had visited

Finally, one night I said, "Geez, Tom! I can't believe how much salt you always put on your food!".

He proceeded without the blink of an eye, "Well, I figure I need the salt to keep my blood pressure high to force the blood through my clogged arteries!"

With that, he happily began chowing down on his salt burgers. In essence, it was true what he said.

Carefully nestling the bag on the passenger's seat, I drove around the building and pulled into a parking spot under some trees. It was May in Pensacola, Florida, hot and humid already. I left the truck idling with the air conditioner on, as I reached into the bag to retrieve the precious contents. Eyeing the bun, I rationalized that it wasn't very big -- probably around 25 carbs -- so I decided to eat the whole thing, although not before sprinkling salt on both items. Not as much as Tom did, but just enough to enhance the flavor. Despite knowing that ketchup is loaded with sugar, I still put a tiny dab on the brown paper napkin to touch with each French fry. Indeed, the burger tasted good, and I was relieved to see the meat was actually thoroughly cooked.

As I ate, I did think that it wasn't good for me, but, hey, once in a while it won't kill you, right? I did consider that the drive space around the building to the spot where we place our orders was kind of narrow, almost like the chute where cattle are herded into the slaughterhouse. Well, basically you are in the slaughterhouse line when going to order most fast food, as it could help you to meet your demise faster. Glancing at the clock, I chowed down the food quickly. I was due for an appointment in 30 minutes. I was very curious what this visit would reveal.

This meeting came about because one of my bosses at my hospital where I work had called me about my schedule. Dr. Nguyen was eating papaya when he called me a few days earlier. Ever since I had discovered I had Type 2 Diabetes on Labor Day in 2017, I had stopped eating any fruit. Oh, I love fruit, any and all of it. However, my Primary Care Physician stated the importance of avoiding fruit "because fruit contains sugar." After that, I would walk through the produce aisles longingly looking at all the beautiful fruit, while sadly thinking of how I'd never be able to enjoy it again. Sometimes, I was so sad about the prohibition of fruit that tears actually welled up in my eyes and trickled down my face. Now -- a few days earlier before my appointment -- Dr. Nguyen, one of the anesthesiologists in charge of our scheduling for the operating room cases each day, was chomping on something as he talked. Kind of annoying to listen to.

"What are you eating?" I inquired.

I could tell he had a smile on his face, when he replied, "I'm eating papaya. You need to go to the Walmart Neighborhood Market right by your house to get some. It's super ripe and delicious!"

Frowning, I responded: "You know I have diabetes, and I can't eat any fruit because it's loaded with sugar!"

He quickly replied, "Yes, you can eat fruit!"

Then back and forth we went: "No, I can't." "Yes, you can." And both of us were sure we were right!

"You know," he said, "in Vietnam everyone is eating white rice three times a day and all kinds of fruit, and there's very few people with diabetes there!"

"If I ate white rice, I'd be in a coma for days," I responded.

I wondered why was it that the Vietnamese can eat tons of white rice; yet, they don't have high rates of diabetes! Remember, my Primary Care Physician kept telling me that carbohydrates and sugars are the main cause of diabetes and to avoid them at all cost. That position was also in my findings online, as I researched Type 2 Diabetes looking for a natural cure.

The next day, I was thinking more about Dr. Nguyen and his juicy papaya. How badly I wished I could be eating a juicy papaya!

Then, impulsively, I reached for my phone and sent him a text message: "I think I'm going to go on a Vietnamese diet and eat all the papaya I want." I sent it as a joke, but part of me wished it were true.

Several minutes later, he sent me a reply: "If you are serious about losing weight and getting rid of diabetes, you need to talk to my sister. She will put on a show for you for an hour and entertain you!"

I was puzzled. Seconds later, my phone was ringing. Dr. Nguyen boomed: "I'll hook you up with my sister if you are really serious!"

"Yes! Hook me up with her," I quickly responded. What does she know?"

"She'll entertain you for an hour. I'll call her to see when you can go over to her house. She lives right near you." A few hours later, he texted me: "She wants to see you on Monday, May 13th at 4 pm., just after you get out of work."

OK. So, the date was set. I didn't know what she could do for me, but, at that point, I didn't see I had any other options. I truly hoped that she could somehow help turn my unhealthy situation around.

Back to the present...I dipped my last French fry into the ketchup and popped it into my mouth. Taking that last sip, I finished the diet Coke, while I gathered up all the food wrappers, stuffing them neatly into the bag. Little did I know that would be my very last burger and fries I would ever eat.

By the time I reached Dr. Nguyen's sister Mimi's house, I already had my daily headache and was feeling pretty sick all over. Even without checking it, I could sense my blood sugar was around 300, not good. I assumed I felt bad, because I chose to eat the whole bun, the carbs I normally did not eat. The truth be told, even without that, I would still be feeling bad. That was my world for over the last two years, every day! The symptoms of Type 2 Diabetes were slowly creeping in, long before I actually discovered I had it. While the symptoms were obvious, I was ignoring them or justifying them with my non-stop lifestyle. The more I read and talked to others with Type 2 Diabetes, I found this to be true for most of the time for others also. As a top tier medical professional, I am embarrassed to say that I ignored so many symptoms for a long time. If this is true in your life, learn from my mistakes and change your life NOW.

Chapter 2. Dismissing Symptoms of Type 2 Diabetes

It was Labor Day 2017 when I discovered I had diabetes. I had diabetic symptoms for many months prior to that day, which I brushed off as due to my crazy and busy professional life. I work full time as a Certified Registered Nurse Anesthetist, which requires that I had to get up by 2:45 am each workday, five days a week.

I'm in the operating room by 5:30 a.m., where I begin my long and stressful day providing anesthesia for one case after another. As an individual on the autism spectrum, my job stresses me far more than any of my colleagues. It is not the actual job of administering anesthesia that is stressful; it is the massive "sensory overload" of that environment.

Bright lights are particularly disturbing to someone who is autistic but also are the sounds from bone saws, hammering, drills, multiple people talking simultaneously, numerous monitors beeping, pungent smells like bone cement, and, almost always, loud music playing. All of that is going on for hours, while anesthesia -- whether general or spinal -- requires staying focused on the patient to provide excellent care. In case you don't know, stress increases cortisol release, which, in turn, increases blood glucose levels.

Fortunately, my job gives me six weeks paid vacation per year. I have used my vacation time to travel around the country giving keynote presentations at autism conferences. I became an autism activist, after discovering that, at the age 50, I am on the autism spectrum.

As a motivational speaker, I have been all over the world, which included being a guest speaker at the United Nations Headquarters in New York City. I am an award-winning author, writing books, guest chapters for other authors' books, articles for magazines, interviews, and blogs. My life is also filled with our rescue animals, grocery shopping, cooking, laundry and managing a household. My husband Abraham is also on the autism spectrum and works full time as well. Given we live on a farm, we have plenty to do.

With all that going on, the extreme exhaustion I gradually began to feel really didn't set off any alarms. When I would get up in the morning, I did notice that I, literally, felt more tired than when I went to bed. I needed to set my alarm for three alarms, five minutes apart. I just could not get up on the first alarm. Finally, after the third one sounded, I would slowly sit up on the side of the bed. It took me another few minutes to be able to get up and walk into the kitchen. My brain would be foggy, and I literally felt like cement was going through my veins instead of blood. Again, I attributed it to my crazy life.

My husband already had coffee brewing, which I desperately needed to help me come to life. Pouring a cup for myself, I would then add a good amount of heavy cream, followed by ten packets of Splenda. Oh my gosh, I can't believe I have shared that very embarrassing tidbit: ten packs of Splenda!

Heck, I've gone this far, so I'll tell you the rest. One of my autistic traits is the need for everything being organized and categorized. In order to use the Splenda, I had to get each little packet and line them up all together, stacked on top of each other, with the front of the packet, correct side up. Not even one could be out of alignment. Then I hold them all at the top to shake them twice to be sure all the powder goes to the bottom of the packets. I then would tear them open at once and pour all the Splenda into the coffee. I never give it a second thought, because that's how I've been doing it forever. One day a co-worker saw me arranging my packets, and she had quite the meltdown. She really flipped out watching me lining them all up so perfectly (much less with how many packets I was using.).

I did start noticing that I was getting blurry vision. I rationalized that, at age fifty-eight, *everybody* needs glasses or, at least those "readers" you get from the grocery store. I even started taking mental inventory of how many co-workers were wearing glasses, most all of whom were, perhaps, twenty years younger than me. So, why would I be so concerned about blurry vision, right? The only thing I did notice was that the blurriness was not consistent. It seemed worse at certain times. But, again, I just brushed it off and didn't focus on it. Then, there was the nausea every morning, when I'd been getting ready for work, which only seemed to occur in the wee hours.

Typical of someone with autism, I have a moderate-to-high level of anxiety, something I've learned to live with throughout my life. Sometimes, if my anxiety gets high, it makes me feel nauseous. So, yet again, I had a rationale for yet another symptom lurking in my life. The nausea was not bad enough to deter me from eating. I considered it mild, just another small problem.

The week before Labor Day 2017, I flew out to Colorado State University in Fort Collins, Colorado. I went there to attend a 70th birthday celebration of another autistic friend, Dr. Temple Grandin. Traveling really takes a toll on me; however, this trip seemed to be worse than others. Throughout the evening I couldn't quench my thirst. I kept making one trip after another to the iced tea dispenser. Earlier that day Temple had taken me out to the farm owned by the university, where her graduate students learn about cattle. I had been out in the sun a lot, so I figured I got dehydrated.

I arrived back at the hotel around 11:00 PM. My husband and our cat had been there all day, and he was looking forward to hearing all about the event. We decided to order room service, so both of us ordered a cheeseburger, fries, and a piece of decadent chocolate fudge cake. We had to get up at 2:00 am for an Uber drive to Denver International Airport to arrive in time for our 6:00 am flight to Atlanta. By the time the food arrived, it was nearly midnight, so we got exactly one hour of sleep that night.

Looking back, I now realize I was teetering on the brink of collapsing into a diabetic coma, which, often, results in death. I was still massively dehydrated, and I ate all that food, including the sugar-laden cake.

When the alarm went off at 2:00 am, I was literally stunned. I felt seriously ill -- like nothing I've ever felt before -- and I was extremely short of breath. I did mention to my husband that I felt sick, but I really didn't want to share how sick I really felt.

The Uber ride that I had scheduled didn't show up, but, fortunately, an Uber driver who was ready to end his shift answered my request to drive the one-and-a-half-hour journey to the airport. After loading all our luggage into the SUV, I sat there in the cramped back seat, where I started thinking that I was going to die from whatever was wrong with me. I did realize that during the whole day before, I did not drink enough, so I was still massively thirsty. My dehydration plus the food I ate the night before were all adding up to a critical situation.

I now know my blood sugar was catastrophically high that morning. All I can tell you is that I truly thought I was going to die. How I didn't is beyond me. Maybe, it was the tough peasant stock I came from, being Czech and Austrian.

The Uber driver, Zach, was just what I needed to help keep me afloat for the drive. He was quite the talker and told one funny story after another. His highlight story was about his grandfather and "Mike, the Headless Chicken." The story was so crazy, I thought he must have made it up!

I recently Googled "Mike, the Headless Chicken" and nearly fainted to see the event actually did happen. Zach had us mesmerized with the bizarre story, enough so to keep me going. I gave him a huge tip once at Denver International Airport. The urge to go to sleep was overwhelmingly strong, but his endless chatter had kept me awake. I had this ominous feeling that, if I went to sleep, I'd never wake up again. I was probably correct.

Once we were through security and seated at our gate, we gravitated to a restaurant with big breakfasts: scrambled eggs, double order of bacon, hash browns, toast slathered with butter and jelly, a large coffee with a ton of half & half and too many packets of Splenda. I want to mention here I had an addiction to Splenda, at least ten packets in every cup of coffee or iced tea. I obviously liked everything super sweet.

All that food, of course, made me feel even more sick. What was I thinking? I did think I was doing the right thing, though, by consuming the huge amount of animal protein. Of course, I didn't have to add the hash browns nor the toast and jelly.

A Nurse Anesthetist I used to work with, Carl, hated to fly with a passion. I thought that to be quite funny, as he spent twenty years in the Navy and had to fly a lot. Carl's motto was, "A chance to fly is a chance to die." Each time I stepped into a plane, I heard Carl's words. So, I justified eating all the carbs I had that morning, because, well, I might not make it anyway. Little did I know, there was a far greater chance of me going down then that 757 in which we were flying.

I finished up the last forkful of food, just in time to board the plane. Once airborne, I could not fight anymore the urge to fall asleep. The next thing I knew the flight attendant was shaking me awake, as we were making our initial descent into Atlanta International Airport. There was still a short layover, then on to the Pensacola International Airport, and, then the ride home. Somehow, I survived all that. Once home, we both went right to sleep and slept about 14 hours until the next morning.

When I woke up, that stunned feeling was still present. Now, I was so thirsty I just could not get enough to drink. I knew I was dehydrated, but I didn't give it a second thought. I was focused on an article I was writing for a magazine, so I sat at the kitchen table all day working on that. I usually don't drink much soda, but there had been a great deal on Fresca diet peach, so I bought some. At the time I figured they'd last for many months, but they did not! I sat, typing away, drinking can after can of the diet soda.

After about the twelfth can, my husband said, "Good grief. I've never seen you drink barely one can of soda, and, now, you just finished a whole case. What's going on?"

Popping yet another can, I started guzzling it down. I simply could not quench my thirst, no matter how fast I was drinking. Still, ashamedly, I still wasn't concerned. Again, I rationalized that, of course. I was thirsty, as my body was simply making up for my dehydrated condition.

Finally, it was early afternoon, and, on one of my many trips to the bathroom, I literally walked into the wall of the doorway leading into the bathroom. I hit it so hard, it took my breath away. That ... that was my wake-up call! *Finally.*

It took that moment for me to realize that there was something seriously wrong with me. While I stood there for a few moments, I suddenly felt like I was going to faint, but I didn't. Waves of nausea were coming, and I, now, had serious blurry vision. I made my way back into the kitchen, holding onto things as I went. My husband, who was washing dishes, turned around to look at me. I saw the panic on his face, as he lurched forward to grab onto me, because I was about to fall.

"What's wrong? What's wrong?" he blurted out.

I finally admitted I was in dire condition. I knew I needed to find out what my blood sugar was. My last blood work was over a year ago or, maybe, even a year and a half. It had been normal at that time.

I somehow mustered the wherewithal to drive to the local pharmacy to purchase a blood glucose monitor. Round trip: 18 minutes. Don't ask what possessed me to drive in that condition. Once home, I immediately pulled everything out and did the finger stick. I watched the little screen, waiting to see my results. It showed 510. Well, of course, I thought, it was only a $35 monitor, so it must be worthless. It couldn't possibly be correct.

I decided to see what my husband Abraham's blood sugars were, in order to test the monitor. I stuck him five times in a row. Each time it showed perfectly normal numbers, like 72 or 81. Then I stuck myself again and touched the little strip onto the tiny drop of blood on my fingertip. 508. There was my answer. Loud and clear. That moment stood still. Diabetes. Type 2 Diabetes. I had it big-time. Oh. My. God.

As a healthcare provider for over 28 years at that time, I constantly saw the reality of the devastating effects of diabetes on patients: the ones coming to the operating room to get arterio-venous shunts for dialysis; the blind ones; the ones coming to get their foot or leg removed because of the gangrene that set in from the serious vascular problems that come with diabetes. All those people flashed through my mind. I was horrified. I sunk into panic mode.

I made my way over to my favorite recliner chair for comfort. So, here I was, a high-level health care professional who has dealt with crisis situations in the operating room my whole life, who now couldn't think of what to do for myself. What a mess. So, what do I do? I texted Dr. Nguyen to tell him my blood glucose is 510 to get his advice, as if I didn't already know I needed to get to the hospital.

Once in the Emergency Room, they started an IV for fluids. My blood sugar was still 510, and my A1C also high at 12.4 After two liters of fluids, they administered eight units of Regular insulin. Then after a total of six liters of fluid, my blood glucose came down to 289. Still too high, they wanted to admit me to the hospital. I didn't want to stay, so I was then discharged to go home, against the recommendation of the ER physician.

The moment I got home, I headed straight to my computer. I began searching for a natural way to cure diabetes. First, I am *extremely* sensitive to medication. Plus, I must confess, I am afraid of most drugs because, they all come with complications, some minor but some more deadly. That's not-to-mention I've seen my share of fatal reactions to drugs in patients over the years. In particular, with one of the top, most widely prescribed diabetes' medications, I saw two patients who began putting out black urine, the sign that their demise was looming near. This particular drug, if used in the presence of dehydration can cause fatal lactic acidosis. That's what those two patients had. That was too close for my liking. This drug even has a Black Box Warning (the most serious warning issued to a drug) regarding the issue of dehydration. Considering I often get dehydrated -- a problem I've had my whole life -- I wasn't really interested in taking this drug or any of them, for that matter.

Four days later I had an appointment with my Primary Care Physician. He spent his usual ten minutes with me, most of which he spent typing away on the computer in the exam room. He gave me the Type 2 Diabetes lecture and handed me several prescriptions: one for Metformin, one for Glipizide, one for Regular insulin, needles, and a statin drug.

Then came the talk about food. There would not have been *any* discussion about food if I had not initiated one. I stated I knew not to eat anything with sugar, which I had already started doing.

"You need to cast the net even wider," he retorted. "Carbohydrates are the main cause of Type 2 Diabetes, so you need to get rid of them, almost totally out of your diet. No more than 50 to 70 grams of carbs per day. And stick to a high protein diet."

And out the door he went.

Chapter 3. Going Through the Stages of Grief

In the weeks that followed, I went into a deep depression. It lasted several months. It knocked me flat. Looking back, I realize I was actually going through the stages of grief – denial, anger, bargaining, depression, and acceptance. I mentioned this to my Primary Care Physician months later, and he made me feel worse by reiterating that patients would rather receive a cancer diagnosis than diabetes, because – as he told me before -- there is no cure for diabetes.

I felt so alone, so overwhelmed, and so defeated. It was extremely difficult not to let my sadness show on my face at work. It probably did, but no one said anything about it. Some days, I'd just burst into tears and curl up on the couch covered with a blanket.

Four months later, while making my next visit to him, my A1C had come down to 8.9, but my daily blood glucose numbers were hovering around 250, typically highest in the early morning. I was following the Keto-type diet, exercising for at least 30 minutes each day, and even was doing some intermittent fasting, also part of the Keto-type diet.

During my endless searches to lower blood sugars, I'd find things such as adding a teaspoon of cinnamon to coffee, which helps lower blood sugar. I read that drinking water with apple cider vinegar could help too. I had that every night before going to bed. I read that eating a whole lemon, skin and all, helped insulin work better. From that information I came up with a crazy shake recipe – some almond milk, a whole lemon, a scoop of whey protein powder, and, yep, you guessed it, ten packets of Splenda! There had to be enough sweetness to override the bitter taste of the lemon peel. It actually did work to some degree, because my blood sugars went from the 300's into the 200's. At least, I felt a little progress was occurring.

I was not taking any of the medication the doctor prescribed. I tried it, but, as I figured would happen, the side effects were too much, which forced me not to go to work. I ended up calling in sick for a whole week, which simply could not go on. I stopped taking everything.

Chapter 4. Searching for a Natural Cure

As I continued my search for a natural cure for Type 2 Diabetes, I looked up the American Diabetes Association website, which basically gave the same information as my Primary Care Physician. I found no references to the whole food plant-based diet, nor did Dr. Neal Barnard's name or his research on Type 2 Diabetes appear. I never came close to what I so desperately needed. It wasn't that I was not trying or that I was not concerned about my health. In fact, the whole diabetes thing was causing me *great* concern, adding yet another layer of anxiety to my already-high level.

My cortisol level was sky high all the time, which affects your blood sugar with higher levels. I felt I was on a downward spiral in which I saw no way of recovery while, all the time, I was eating my high protein diet. Then, in October of 2018, I flew to Washington D.C. to speak at the Federal Communications Commission for "National Employees with Disabilities Month." From the stress of the trip, my blood sugar soared up farther again.

I knew at my follow-up visit with my Primary Care Physician that I was not going to make him happy. I knew that he was fed up with me because I would not take the pills. I was just as unhappy with him for not having any answers for my continued requests for an alternative cure for diabetes.

He did suggest I go for bariatric surgery for a gastric by-pass. I nearly hit the floor when he said that. Indeed, my weight was high -- very high -- like 298 pounds to be exact. However, I have provided anesthesia for hundreds of those cases, so I know exactly the mechanics of the operation and how it affects the body and what can go wrong. I'd rather be overweight than risk my health and my life for that. I also knew that the reason he suggested gastric by-pass surgery is that it pretty much cures a person of their Type 2 Diabetes. In the first part of the small intestine, where fats are absorbed, that portion is cut away from the stomach; thus, it is no longer connected to the stomach. After the surgery, you are only able to eat a very tiny amount of food at any given meal. Any fats that are consumed are poorly absorbed. In addition to weight loss, insulin resistance disappears. It might sound enticing; however, there are risks of this type of surgery. In a study from 1995 to 2004, out of 16,683 patients who underwent bariatric gastric by-pass surgery, there were 440 deaths related to the surgery, because of things like pulmonary embolism, heart attacks, and sepsis.[2] I am providing you a good site to read about all the risks associated with bariatric surgery.[3] Needless to say, I wasn't interested in signing up for the surgery.

Since I mentioned the weight issue, it's something I have struggled with my entire life. I have tried practically every diet that I could find. All of them. Weight Watchers, Jenny Craig, TOPS, Atkins, South Beach, the list goes on. I'm a big girl, even without the excess weight. I am 5'9" and big boned. I have always been around horses and worked on a farm. How long do you think I would last on tiny portions of food that I had to measure out? I don't do well when I'm hungry. I am the true definition of "Hangry," for sure! Not one of those diets could I stick with or worked for me.

I can remember seeing a co-worker at lunch one day, who had just started one of these diets. I don't know how they package their food nowadays, but, back then, some foods came in tiny silver cans. When she popped open the lid, it sounded and looked like a can of cat or dog food. To me, it smelled the same too. The frustrating thing was that I really did not eat much junk food, if any at all. I did eat a lot of meat, chicken, pork, and dairy products. I don't do well counting calories, weighing portion sizes, keeping track of points, making charts or anything else when it comes to food. That sends me into a tailspin. I just want to eat and not spend time obsessing over it or writing things down. I wondered why there couldn't be a way to eat that could fulfil my dreams of just eating whatever I wanted, whenever I wanted, but still lose weight? At least I could dream about it, right?

My A1C was back up to 12.1 at the appointment right after the Washington D.C. trip. My fasting blood sugar was 245, when the bloodwork was evaluated prior to the visit. The doctor tolerated me that day, prescribing more diabetes' drugs, Januvia and Victoza, which I had no intention to take, because of my reaction to drugs, but I took the prescriptions and left his office. I am sure he knew I had no intentions of taking them as well. It's not that I set out to be an obnoxious patient, I simply wanted a solution for treating things *naturally.* I realize medications can be extremely helpful and even lifesaving, but medication comes with side effects, as I have mentioned earlier. Most are mild, but some are deadly. It might only be a tiny percentage of patients that are affected with the serious side effects, but to those people and their families, it can be a pretty big deal, especially if it ends their lives or causes some catastrophic effects. As a result, there are more and more individuals looking for natural remedies, how to become more mindful, and simply to have better health and a better life naturally. It seems to me, if there is something which can be successfully treated or reversed without drugs, my view is you are safer to go that route.

Chapter 5. Getting Fired by My Primary Care Physician

It was March 2019, and I was due for another follow up visit. Walking into the fancy, upscale medical center where my Primary Care Physician had his office, I pretty much knew what was about to happen. Once in the exam room, the nurse came in with a release form to sign. It was regarding the new Google Glasses the doctor would be wearing. The glasses would be recording both audio and visual of each patient encounter. It would then transcribe the voice recording and relay that and the video footage to a central location as a permanent record. That would allow him to see more patients by not having to take the time to dictate the visit after each patient.

Between him typing away at lightning speed on his computer when I'd talk and looking through his Google Glasses, I was even more stressed out. To him, the Google Glasses signified a faster, easier way to see a higher volume of patients each day. To me, it seemed that I was like a cow in a line-up in a cattle chute, disconnected from my physician. He announced that he didn't feel comfortable continuing as my doctor, because I was a high-risk patient who was non-compliant. On one hand, I could see that from his perspective. On the other hand, I thought, subsequently, he should have known about the whole food plant-based diet and should have offered that to me as my very first option of treatment for Type 2 Diabetes. Like most physicians, they are not taught about nutrition in medical school, so he probably didn't know about it.

How ironic. Non-compliant. For over a year and a half, I was desperately searching for a natural way to cure my diabetes. I'd ask him each time I was there, thinking, perhaps, he might have learned something I hadn't found. Nothing. Over and over again, he'd write out prescriptions or tell me to go get an invasive, dangerous surgery or procedure. Initially, it was Metformin, Glipizide, and insulin. Then, he tried to get me to take Januvia and then Victoza.

When it comes to pharmaceuticals, the first thing anyone should do is to read about possible serious side effects. All I needed to see is things like "acute pancreatitis, hemorrhagic and necrotizing pancreatitis sometimes resulting in death," and, yep, that did it for me.

Once he even made the comment, half joking, "If you don't take these pills, I won't get paid!" The tales of Big Pharma are plentiful, but I will refrain from that focus now.

You might be wondering what exactly I was eating for that year and a half after getting diagnosed. The main goal was always aimed at eating as much protein as possible in each meal. Breakfast was often scrambled eggs, ham, with, maybe some broccoli. After I discovered that lemons increase insulin functioning, I was having the shake with whey protein powder for breakfast. Lunch would consist of cold cuts like ham, turkey, some cheese, or baked chicken or pork chops. Dinner would be something like Sockeye salmon, which I'd spread on some mayonnaise and sprinkle on grated parmesan cheese before baking it. More broccoli, asparagus, or sautéed cabbage. I never ate that much protein in my life, until I received the diabetes' diagnosis and instructions from my Primary Care Physician.

When I got up from the chair to leave the exam room, I didn't say a word to him. There was nothing to say. He was done with me, and I was done with him just the same.

I made my way out to my truck and burst into tears. I didn't know what else to do. I truly wanted to get my health back and the diabetes under control. I was totally lost and at wit's end.

A week later I received a Certified Letter from that Primary Care Physician officially stating he had discharged me as his patient.

I realized I needed to look for a new Primary Care Physician, because you need one as your gateway to specialists, if needed, or for any unforeseen circumstances. I began looking into finding one who was open to incorporating natural ways to healing, like a naturopathic physician. If I was living in another part of the country, I may have had better luck. Naturopathic physicians aren't known to flock to Pensacola, FL. I learned from talking to a lady I met that her doctor was open-minded and seemed to focus on wellness, so I asked her for his name and made an appointment. I was hoping he might be an improvement over the last one, possibly offering some ideas for a natural way to bring down blood sugar and increase insulin functioning. My appointment with him was for May 22, 2019.

There was a six-week period of time from getting fired from the "Google Glasses Doc" to my other most fateful day, which was May 13, 2019. That was my appointment with Mimi, which would change everything.

I was obsessed with finding a path to natural healing. Each time I'd do a search on the Internet, I used the key words "naturally cure Type 2 Diabetes," "foods that heal Type 2 Diabetes," "Food remedies for Type 2 Diabetes," and "how to cure diabetes."

No matter how these phrases were entered, I received the same results. There were plenty of times I cried myself to sleep at night, knowing my life would be over far sooner, because of my uncontrolled diabetes. I thought about it morning, noon, and night.

Each time I had a patient with diabetes with one or more of its devastating side effects, I would become hysterical inside, knowing that would be me one day. I felt trapped inside a body that I saw as failing me. *Why me? Why did I have to get this progressive disease? Why does anyone have to get it?* I kept asking those questions over and over.

Chapter 6. Finding Answers: The Turning Point

As I pulled into Mimi's driveway, her husband was outside picking blueberries off a bush in their front garden. She heard my vehicle and came out through the garage to greet me. They both led the way into the house, removing their shoes on a mat in the garage just before entering inside. They motioned for me to do likewise. That is traditional Vietnamese, which I already knew from visiting the Vietnamese Temple nearby in the past.

Once inside, Mimi's "entertainment" began. She and I both sat at the kitchen island, where her laptop sat, along with several books, and a bowl filled with tomatoes and various vegetables, and some I realized were unrecognizable. I presumed those were from the Vietnamese market, where I later learned you can find exotic fruits and vegetables you will never see at traditional grocery stores.

Mimi is an Emergency Department physician at the same hospital where I work. She's been there over sixteen years. She graduated from Johns Hopkins University School of Medicine with her degree as an emergency medicine physician.

Climbing onto the high island chair, Mimi turned her laptop towards me. Her brother had already informed her about my diabetes' situation.

She began, "Have you ever heard of the whole food plant-based diet?" Furrowing my brows, I replied, "No, I'm not familiar with it." She was quickly scrolling up and down on the screen looking for something specific. Looking very intently at me, Mimi began 'the show.'

"Have you ever heard of The China Study? The book is based on the China-Cornell-Oxford Study. Dr. T. Colin Campbell was one of the study's directors. This study examined the link between consumption of animal products and chronic illnesses, such as coronary heart disease, diabetes, breast cancer, prostate cancer, and bowel cancer. The authors concluded that people who eat a predominantly whole food plant-based diet and avoid animal products and processed foods will avoid, reduce, or reverse the development of many diseases. It basically means 'If it has a face or a mother, you don't eat it!'"

I sat in silence as she continued, "Have you ever seen a documentary called Forks Over Knives?" Suddenly my mind came to life.

"Yes!" I blurted out!

Mimi then continued: "You can reverse your diabetes by following a whole food plant-based diet. No drugs. Just eat this way, and you can turn it around."

My initial thoughts were to wonder why I had not come across any of this during my year and a half of searching for a natural cure for diabetes. Many years earlier, I actually did see that documentary. In fact, one of the people in it had a very unusual name that I somehow remembered.

"Isn't that the one where there's a physician named Dr. Caldwell Esselstyn?" I asked.

Looking surprised, Mimi answered "Yes!"

My mind was suddenly flooded with scenes from that documentary. What I remembered most was how I watched it, thinking it would be impossible to get enough protein if all you did was eat plants. I also recalled the many things I had going on in my life at the time, which consumed me to the point I wasn't open to new ideas or suggestions.

Then came the moment that would change my life. "Have you ever heard of Dr. Neal Barnard? He's the one who focuses on reversing diabetes," Mimi inquired.

I froze. My mind raced back in time. Right then, Mimi reached over to the stack of books at the end of the counter. Selecting one, she handed it to me. It was a very emotional moment for me. It was Dr. Barnard's book, *Dr. Neal Barnard's Program for Reversing Diabetes Without Drugs.* Many years earlier, around 2006, my mom saw Dr. Barnard on a popular medical show, and she tried to get me to start Dr.

Barnard's plan. At that time, I was taking care of both her and my dad. I took care of them until they died in 2013 and 2014, respectively. I was working full time and was overwhelmed with caring for them, both physically and emotionally.

Even more, each day there was a new "diet of the day" on TV medical shows and in the top magazines. It seemed like just another fad, so I didn't listen. I did not have diabetes at the time, but my mom saw Dr. Barnard's program as an extremely healthy way of eating. She asked me to get a copy of his book, which I did right away. She read that book, cover to cover, and was literally begging me to go on it with her. She always referred to him as Dr. Neal Bernard, with the emphasis on the 'Nard' part, so it sounded like Ber-NARD.

She also made lots of comments on how handsome he was, so I just figured she was enthralled with him. I wasn't interested in any of it at the time. I now realize that it just wasn't the right time in my life to start eating that way.

As a result, I want to help others make it the "right time now" in *their* lives so they can take charge of their health for a better life.

As I sat at that kitchen table with this ER doc with a passion for the plant-based diet, it hit me like a ton of bricks, no, cinderblocks. Yes! This is the answer I've been looking for all this time.

I asked her, why did NONE of these physicians, especially Dr. Neal Barnard, nor the whole food plant-based diet *ever* come up during my endless research for a natural way to cure or reverse Type 2 Diabetes?

I was so overwhelmed with emotions I burst out crying. Mimi quickly reached over to rest her hand on my arm. "But why are you crying," she asked.

"Probably, if my mom and I had gone on this diet all those years ago, she would still be alive today," I replied between sobbing. I could not even allow my mind to go there. I'm sure many people have something happen in their lives that they wish they could go back in time to do something different, to prevent a devastating outcome. I should have, would have, could have.

That sadness was overcome with the thought that, now, I had the answer I had been relentlessly searching for – the whole food, plant-based diet to reverse my diabetes without drugs.

I was extremely grateful to her for taking that time with me. It was that fateful meeting that flipped on the switch in my brain. All that knowledge I had all along, but it was hidden away until now.

As I left Mimi's home that day, with Dr. Barnard's book tightly clutched to my chest, I went cold-turkey and *immediately* started on his plan. Well, I guess I'd better re-phrase that to "cold-Tofu!"

I didn't have the necessary food initially, so I started out the next day with nothing but a head of broccoli. I had a raging headache that I suffered with all day at work. Yet, I was determined to stick with the diet, so I suffered through that headache.

Don't do what I did in this regard! I will inform you on how to be fully prepared, so you can start in a positive way.
Dr. Barnard outlines an initial program that helps a novice to approach this new way of eating in a three-week time frame. This allows you to gently ease into it.

This plant-based diet has endless, beautiful meals to make, which are not only life-changing but delicious. Beginning does take a re-structuring of your lifestyle. However, the rewards are worth it.

Within days I began feeling dramatically better. By the end of the first week, my blood glucose levels were dramatically coming down. By the fourth week my blood glucose levels were down in the 80's! Even an hour after a meal, I'd see 87 on my Accucheck monitor! I felt *spectacular!* I had energy like I couldn't believe: no more exhaustion, no shortness of breath.

Within a year, I had lost 70 pounds. I am fully committed to continuing this new way of life. I will share that my husband also started this journey with me, and he has also lost 70 pounds! He didn't have any other health issues.

The whole food plant-based diet isn't just for reversing diabetes. It can reverse heart disease, inflammatory diseases, autoimmune diseases, and, even, some forms of cancer. It's also a great, healthy way to lose weight!

I am eternally grateful to Dr. Barnard and all he has done for those with Type 2 Diabetes. He gave me back my life. I truly felt like I was ready to die; now, I'm full of vitality and have a new outlook on life. Without any further delay, let's get you going on your new way of eating.

Part 2:

How to Start Your Own Journey to Your Best Health

Chapter 7. Starting on a Plant-Based Lifestyle

One of my learning objectives is to enable you to better understand the science of Type 2 Diabetes. I won't go into elaborate details, but I certainly will direct you to where you can read about it in greater depth. Through this information you will see that medications are only dealing with the symptoms and not the root cause. The best way to address the root cause is to get your body healthy on a cellular level. The *best* way to do this is through the powers of a whole food plant-based diet.

Recently, I attended a conference on this topic, where one of the presenters showed a slide that pretty much spells it out. It was a cartoon of two people with mops frantically mopping up water that was pouring onto the floor from a running sink. Instead of turning off the sink and solving the problem, they kept mopping up the water spilling over the side of the sink, never addressing the real issue.

The same holds true for Type 2 Diabetes. Medications are prescribed to deal with the high blood glucose levels, but no one addresses how to turn off the problem in the first place. Until now. Dr. Bernard shows us how we can turn off that diabetes' "sink" by eating a whole food plant-based diet.

According to the World Health Organization there are over 422 million people around the world with diabetes. At least 85-90% are Type 2. It is estimated that, if the current trends continue, by 2025 there will be over 700 million adults worldwide affected by diabetes. This number has nearly quadrupled since 1980, when 108 million people were affected with the disease.[4]

In another study by researchers at the University of Gottingen, Harvard T.H. Chan School of Public Health, "the world faces a substantial economic burden from diabetes – about $1.3 trillion, or 1.8% of the global gross domestic product (GDP)." This was published on April 26, 2017 in *The Lancet Diabetes & Endocrinology*. The new study "incorporated not only the direct costs of the disease, such as expenditures for insulin, testing strips, and treatment, but also indirect costs representing production shortfalls due to illness and premature death, which account for nearly 35% of the total economic burden."[5]

I have experienced firsthand the challenges of transitioning to the whole food plant-based diet. I'm not just telling you how or what to do, I'm sharing what I learned that you can use as a guide to begin the journey yourself. I've been there and done that. Now, I'm sharing with you, so you can *try this!*

If you have Type 2 Diabetes and want to reverse what *will* become a progressive disease, please know I'm writing this from my heart. It would be a terrible thing if I simply enjoyed the fruits of my journey and keep it to myself.

When I met Dr. Neal Barnard in Oakland, California, at the Plantrician International Plant-Based Healthcare Conference, I asked him a burning question. I was literally jumping up and down in my seat when I asked, "What can I do to help others with diabetes?"
"The worst thing you could do is to not do anything! he replied. "You are a success story and sharing your story will inspire others to follow."

I know he is right. I must get this message out, so others will learn about the power of a whole food plant-based diet. This includes individuals with diabetes as well as their physicians. After reading all this, you might decide it's not for you, but I'm hoping you will at least try a 21-Day Challenge! Ray, who works in the produce aisle at my grocery store, told me that being a vegan is "the best life insurance policy you could ever get." Ray talked about his daughter and her family, also vegans. He shared photos with me about what his daughter gives her little boy as a snack: a slice of pumpernickel toast with a cut-up banana on it sprinkled with a wisp of cinnamon. Her child is now used to healthy snacks. This is a way of life for anyone who is ready to make a positive change, a permanent change and, in the process, dramatically improve their health.

Here's a good comparison. Imagine you were given a brand-new vehicle, something exotic like a Lamborghini. Would you try to run it with kerosene, which is not the proper fuel for it, or would you want to put in the best quality fuel to enable maximum performance and longevity?

This holds true for the human body as well. We are all given a complex and fascinating body for which we supposedly should care for. Don't you want to enable it to perform at peak levels and become the best you possibly can be? You can extend its "warranty?"

In the operating room, it is not uncommon to see patients that are 12 years old and weigh 250 pounds. The parents will say, "Johnny will only eat mac and cheese and hotdogs." Well, Johnny isn't going to the grocery store by himself. The parents are the enablers to his condition. They are sending Johnny down a path to diabetes, heart disease, and other serious health conditions that could be avoided. There are plenty of reasons why you should pay attention to what you eat. Most people are living hectic lives, between work, family, friends, and obligations. There's little time left of your day.

Unfortunately, what's the quick and easy way to get food in your belly and for your family? The easy answer: highly processed foods that are available in the grocery store or your favorite fast food restaurant where you don't even have to get out of your vehicle. Just drive up and order burgers and fries, fried chicken, barbeque. The sky's the limit. It's all convenient and tasty, but there's one *HUGE* problem.

All of it compromises our health. Other than heartburn or some temporary response with such foods, you won't see the bad effects until later in life. Meanwhile, it will be lurking around, silently inside your body, insidiously doing damage. Often, when we get sick or have some kind of injury or illness, many of us will start Googling to find what we can do to help our body heal.

Instead of waiting for disaster to occur, we need to consider this: food is medicine. Good food. More specifically, a whole food plant-based diet. When you realize that what you eat can be medicine for your body, everything begins to change. You will become in charge of your body and your health. You will start to make better choices about what and how to eat, in order to make the best decisions for your own well-being. The title of this book, *A Food Revolution: How A Plant Based Lifestyle Can Win the Global War on Diabetes, Obesity, and Heart Disease* sounds like some elaborate task force project. Yet, it's quite a simple solution. The remedy for these dire illnesses is right in front of everyone. It is all the foods that naturally grow from our earth: the grains, legumes, vegetables, and fruits. Yes, they're all those beautiful, colorful plants that generated the saying, "Eat the rainbow every day!" That means you should include many colors in your diet, because they can ensure you're getting enough fiber, vitamins, minerals, antioxidants, and the like, to help to protect against illness, bone density loss, digestive problems, and weight management. It is all in the food that grows naturally from the earth. It's nothing processed. Simple. Pure. Honest.

There is no pill that can rival the power of the whole food plant-based diet. I have personally experienced this phenomenon, and I can speak with total confidence that it is nothing short of a miracle. There are endless delicious recipes to make that are quick and easy. There are not any potentially lethal side effects of this way of eating. There are no Black Box Warnings (like on medications.) Not to sound totally negative regarding drugs -- because they can be lifesaving in some situations -- drugs can also be unnecessary or even harmful in other situations.

The greatest task is educating not only those with diabetes but, also, the physicians who are on the frontlines of healthcare.

In 1985, Dr. Neal Barnard founded the Physician's Committee for Responsible Medicine (*pcrm.org*). It combines the expertise of over 12,000 physicians combined with the dedicated actions of over 175,000 members in the United States and around the world.

As stated on the pcrm.org website, "Our efforts are dramatically changing the way doctors treat chronic diseases such as diabetes, heart disease, obesity, and cancer. By putting prevention over pills, doctors are empowering their patients to take control of their own health."

A recent poll of physicians in Washington, D.C. found that 73% of physicians felt nutrition counseling should be provided to patients; yet, only 15% felt prepared to do it.

In support of the Continuing Nutrition Education Amendment Act of 2019, Dr. Barnard testified about the importance of the bill at a Washington, D. C. Council hearing. This bill is calling for continuing education on nutrition for health care providers by providing information which would enable them to incorporate nutrition counseling into their practice.

Fruits, vegetables, legumes, and whole grains each have very specific, powerful nutrients. They contain protein, vitamins, minerals, phytonutrients, antioxidants, and many critical factors to enable the human body to function at its maximum capacity.

Imagine what would happen if you *only* ate these foods. How would your body respond? I can tell you from my personal experience that your body will begin to function like nothing you've ever experienced before. And, the best part, it is that you don't have to wait months or years to begin feeling the positive effects. You will begin to feel the difference within *days.*

Hippocrates, a Greek physician (c. 460-c.370 BC), is considered one of the most outstanding figures in the history of medicine. He is often referred to as the "Father of Medicine" in recognition of his lasting contributions to the field of medicine and founder of the Hippocratic School of Medicine.[6] One of his most popular phrase was "Let thy food be thy medicine and medicine be thy food," which is used to emphasize the importance of nutrition to prevent or cure disease.

Chapter 8. Let's Talk About Animal Products

Animal products of food include meat, chicken, pork, fish, eggs, milk, butter, yogurt, and cheese. There is a large and ever-growing amount of research-backed evidence that animal products are unhealthy food choices. It's much too involved to go into depth for the scope of this book, so I have provided a list of articles and research papers to verify this statement at the end of this book.

This might sound a bit strange; however, I feel compelled to say it. For seven years I worked at one of the biggest organ transplant university hospitals in America. I did the anesthesia for the different organ transplants, such as livers, kidneys, hearts, and lungs. The patients who were the recipients receiving the organ transplants had to take a myriad of drugs - - often called "the anti-rejection drugs" -- for the rest of their lives.

When an organ from one human being is transplanted into another, the recipient's body recognizes the organ as a foreign object. This is because the person's immune system detects that the antigens in the cells of the organ are different or not "matched." "Mismatched organs" or organs that are not matched closely enough can trigger a blood transfusion reaction or transplant rejection.

So, why am I telling you this? Well, now that I'm totally off ALL animal products, all the inflammation is gone from my body. I started thinking . . . It's almost as if ingesting animal flesh is akin to receiving an organ from another body. You are eating flesh from a living creature. It is foreign to the human body.

The meat takes about five days to reach the grocery store from the time the animal was killed. Then the consumer buys the product, then maybe another day before they prepare it. From the time you eat that meat, chicken, fish, or whatever it is, that dead carcass is now inside your body for at least one to two days, possibly longer. Then, because people are eating animal products at most every meal, that means there is a constant level of that "foreign" object in the body most of the time. In response, our body is rejecting it by reacting with chronic inflammation throughout your body.

I can feel the dramatic difference of not having inflammation. Aside from reversing Type 2 Diabetes, hypertension, and a 70-pound weight loss, all the aches and pains I had for years throughout my body went away. So has the trigger finger on my left hand. That was so bad, I was already trying to figure out when I could get the surgery, to fit it into my hectic schedule. Now, I don't need to worry about that any longer. The trigger finger is long gone. My hand and fingers function completely normally now, as if I never had it. That's better than any surgery could have ever been!

When I was 21, I ruptured a disc in my lumbar spine in a horse accident. Ever since then, for years, I've had stinging and burning in certain areas on my left outer leg. That's also gone! Wow! All of these miraculous changes came about from the plant-based lifestyle! Keep in mind, I have not deviated from the plant-based way of eating: not even on holidays, nothing. It might sound impossible, but my motivation is sustained from the incredible results I am enjoying. Food that I used to eat and crave now makes me sick at the thought of it and, even worse, the sight of it. Why? Because now I know just how sick it used to make me feel.

On the contrary, when I walk into a produce aisle, my eyes light up and I'm singing inside, because I know how great all the fruits and vegetables make me feel. Your taste buds change very rapidly as well, which also removes cravings for things you used to eat.

Dr. Neal Barnard's book *Reversing Diabetes Without Drugs* is what saved my life. I will be referring to many points in that book. Dr. Barnard and his team conducted a series of research studies first with Georgetown University and George Washington University in Washington, D.C., which led to a new approach to diabetes, tested and proven. This evidence now allows many individuals with diabetes to take control of their health. Seen as a progressive disease, Type 2 Diabetes typically is treated with one or more medications to delay the inevitable decline. Instead, from Dr. Barnard's research, people are now able to improve their health dramatically by decreasing their blood sugar, lowering cholesterol levels and blood pressure; decreasing weight; increasing their insulin sensitivity and their energy, and reduction or elimination of medications. [7]

How is this possible? A change of your diet is the key to this outcome. Following a whole food plant-based diet causes a fundamental change in the body itself. In his book, Dr. Barnard states it is "specifically, the body's ability to respond to insulin, the sugar-storing hormone that is dysfunctional in diabetes. This diet change is powerful enough to boost insulin sensitivity and bring blood sugar under better control. We can help the body's own insulin properly work again by directly addressing – and improving – the cells' sensitivity to it, which is the key issue in Type 2 Diabetes." This was based on his research study, which was published in *Preventive Medicine* in 1999. He further goes on to say, "even when the disease has evolved to the point of serious complications, it is not too late for marked improvements to occur." [8]

Dr. Barnard conducted a new research trial starting in 2003, with the support of the National Institutes of Health. He compared his diet guidelines against those of the American

Diabetes Association at the time. The results concluded that Barnard's program "controlled blood sugar three times more effectively than the ADA diet and also accelerates weight loss, lowers cholesterol, and has dramatic benefits for the heart and improves blood pressure. This allows individuals to take charge of their lives and return to health and vigour." [9]

The key to this diet is in avoiding all animal products. When there are no animal products in the diet, there is not a single drop of animal fat. Taking this concept a step farther, eliminating *all* oils ensures no fat from them as well. So, you ask, what is the deal on fats? I'm going to give you a very simple explanation of what fat has to do with Type 2 Diabetes.

You often hear the term "insulin resistance," which is when your body is resistant to the insulin and does not work correctly. Instead, research has shown that fat within cells is what is blocking insulin from entering the cell membrane with the glucose molecules.

Dr. Barnard best describes this as the cells being "gummed up," like a lock with gum in it, which obviously prevents the "key," in this case the insulin molecule carrying a glucose molecule, from entering the cell. When you eliminate animal products from the diet, there is no fat entering the cells, which alters the fat build-up within the cells. Once this begins happening, the insulin can once again gain access to transporting glucose out of the bloodstream and into the cells where it belongs.[10]

To read about it in much more detail, refer to Dr. Barnard's book *Reversing Diabetes Without Drugs.*

I strongly recommend that healthcare providers try this diet for themselves. Not only will it give them the perspective to share with their patients, it will also help achieve optimal health for themselves. After all, this lifestyle isn't just to reverse diabetes, hypertension, inflammatory diseases or, even, cancer, it acts to *prevent* these disease processes from occurring in the first place. Elite athletes – like Venus Williams (tennis); Lewis Hamilton (Formula 1); Scott Jurek (Ultramarathon); Megan Duhamel (2018 Winter Gold Medal Figure Skating); Barny du Plessis (bodybuilding); Patrik Baboumian (Strongman); Alex Morgan (Women's Soccer); and Ruth Heidrich (83-year-old Ironman Triathlete) -- are using this diet to enable them to perform at their maximum capacity. That should tell you something.

So, remember, avoid ALL animal products and ADDED OILS should be eliminated, as these are the fats that raise insulin resistance!

Chapter 9.   Where Will I Get My Protein?

One thing that people ask right away.   Where will I get protein?   This is a whole topic in itself, including people's addiction to protein, which they consider to be animal protein. To first answer the question, your protein will come from the whole grains, legumes, vegetables, and, even fruits.   What? Protein from grains? Vegetables? What?? That's impossible, you are thinking.

I've been an equestrienne most of my life and rode both open jumpers and dressage.   The horses used for these disciplines are huge, powerful animals.   For a horse to be able to jump over an obstacle that's six-feet-high and six-feet-wide takes incredible strength.   What does a horse eat? Hay and grain. Carrots and apples as treats.   So, these great big powerful creatures are eating a whole food plant-based diet.

You also need less protein than what you think you need. As a medical professional, I need to state that you should first consult with your physician before embarking on this diet and/ or any exercise program, to be sure it is safe for you.

There is a great book you should read: *Proteinaholic: How Our Obsession with Meat is Killing Us and What We Can Do About It* by Garth Davis, M.D.

If you are currently taking prescription medications for diabetes, you will need to work with your physician as you embark on the whole food plant-based diet. You will need to have your medications adjusted as you progress and, hopefully, you'll be able to discontinue them at some point. If you stick with this program you will begin to see your blood sugar numbers come down, as well as the numbers on your scale. Your blood sugar will start coming down within *days* of starting this plan, so you will need to check your blood sugar more frequently. I was checking mine literally every 1-2 hours from the time I'd get up until I went to bed. Even checked it during the night! When I set out to reverse my diabetes, I had that goal on my radar. As I started dropping pounds, it was an added bonus.

I was eating whatever I wanted, whenever I wanted, and I felt full and satisfied. There was never another diet I ever tried that would fit this description.

Chapter 10. The First Step: Gutting Out the Fridge

When I arrived home on May 13th, 2019 from Mimi's house, I knew what had to be done *immediately*: gut out the refrigerator of every animal product inside of it. I knew I must get rid of every animal product in the refrigerator and freezer. Yup. Pull over the trash can and get going. Clear out EVERYTHING that is an animal product – meat, chicken, pork, fish, milk, butter, eggs, cheese, yogurt, cream cheese, ice cream.   This includes foods that contain any animal products as ingredients. A bit later, I'll talk more about learning to read labels on *everything*. It seems shocking to do this, but if you are serious about reversing your diabetes, you do not want any of this available.   There is no point to have temptations available in the house, so be sure they are not there.   After a few weeks, several things will happen: your taste buds will change, and, when you start feeling so much better, that, it will be your motivating force.

As I began clearing out the shelves of my refrigerator, I will admit it was an emotional experience. My husband and I were planning a celebration dinner that coming weekend. All the items for a very fancy meal were already stocked in the fridge and freezer. I started with the "easy" stuff.... extricating the eggs, butter, yogurt, milk, and cheese. Clunk, clunk, clunk as each one hit the bottom of the trash can. I sighed as I'd grab another item. Then came the tough part. Out came several New York Strip steaks, and then, the worst of all. Once a year, we treat ourselves to several pounds of Alaskan King Crab legs. They were, in fact, the biggest I'd ever seen. As I held that bag, I stopped. I looked at my husband, then looked back at the bag. I was envisioning the sweet, succulent, delicate meat hidden inside those huge orange shells. I gulped. I asked myself a question right then. *Why am I doing this?* In my mind I wanted to put those Alaskan King Crab legs right back into the freezer. But in my heart, I knew I wanted to get healthy and live. I let out a big sigh. Still not taking my eyes off the package, I softly said, "Why don't we take all these steaks and crab legs across the street to Richard and Melody?"

Very matter of fact, Abraham replied, "why do you want to inflict inflammation on *them?*"

I threw the crab legs into the trash with deliberate force. "You are right. We don't want this anymore for ourselves. We can't give it to anyone." At that moment I felt empowerment. I knew I was taking control of my health and my life.

Once the refrigerator is cleansed, next head to your pantry. Get rid of anything containing animal products and oils. Olive oil, coconut oil, avocado oil, canola oil, *all* oils. Oils are a processed food, and they cause inflammation in your body, in particular, the lining of your heart, the endothelium. [11, 12]

I realize this all seems difficult to believe, because you read that olive oil is heart healthy, and we are constantly bombarded with information promoting meat, dairy, eggs, olive oil, and coconut oil. You will come to learn these are marketing strategies by the industries promoting their products. Here is an example. The meat industry has people believing that real men eat meat.

There's a new documentary, *The Game Changers,* which features Arnold Schwarzenegger addressing this very matter. Watch this trailer to see him talk about the marketing vs. reality factor of the need to eat meat.[13]

Finally, the mission was complete. All animal products were successfully removed from the refrigerator. including even those things that contained an animal product in the ingredient list on the label. It is critical to learn the importance and skill of reading labels on all food products. Manufacturers are very skilled at using ingredients that you may not understand, which can trick you. I will discuss this shortly.

Now remember, I was eating a Keto-type diet for nearly two years after discovering I have Type 2 Diabetes, advice that had been on given by my Primary Care Physician. Thus, the refrigerator was stocked with mostly animal products!

By the time it was all said and done, the only remaining item left in the refrigerator was broccoli: one very lonely head of broccoli sitting on the shelf. It was nearly 8 p.m., too late for a trip to the grocery store.

For breakfast and lunch the next day, we both had broccoli, which was not much, as we had to split it into four portions for our breakfast and lunch. I ended up with a raging headache by mid-morning from hardly eating. And, of course, there was the coffee issue. I love coffee, just one cup a day, but I sure enjoy it. But…. uh…. yikes. I love it loaded with heavy cream and that obscene number of packets of Splenda, 10. That morning I had to drink it black. I didn't have any almond or soymilk, and I couldn't continue with the Splenda. I'll talk about artificial sweeteners in a bit. It was a very pitiful morning indeed. But I wasn't backing out. Not in a million years. I was determined to get rid of diabetes once and for all.

After I finished work for the day, I went shopping for the proper food items to begin the whole food plant-based diet.

Given my experience, however, I now need to explain something. In Dr. Barnard's book, he advises you to do a "test drive" before starting a plant-based diet. Indeed, habits aren't easy to change, and that period of time for planning ahead allows the transition to go more smoothly and successfully.

First, he suggests you look over recipes and new foods suggested in his book to get an idea of what you can begin eating. As long as it fits within the guidelines, then start figuring out a meal plan. Then he talks about setting up a three-week period, actually to begin the diet with 100% commitment. During that time, you must stay true to the food intended or else you won't see the change that will happen.

That was the only thing in Dr. Barnard's book that I disregarded, simply because I was in a dire situation where every second counted. I must also say this – by immediately going plant-based -- I began seeing and feeling results within *days*, which let me know I was on the correct path. Had I taken the test drive route, it would have delayed my improvements from starting immediately.

It is totally up to you as to which path to choose. This was simply my personal choice. I was in a dire situation and saw no choice but to start at 100%, instantly. Dr. Barnard's plan is more likely to get you to transition successfully because, by planning well in advance, you will know what you will be eating, and you can purchase the foods you need to kick-off that 21-day "trial." My only hope is that whichever route you take, it gets you on this journey as soon as possible for your best life ever!

I'd like to add something which might seem unusual. Throughout my entire life, I've been using "visualization" to achieve everything I have accomplished, from everyday little things to getting a flight in an F-15 fighter jet. I used that same visualization to help myself go plant-based, never looking back. It is a very simple -- yet powerful – tool.

Visualization is a mental technique that uses your imagination, mental images, and the power of thoughts to develop a laser-focus, to do what is necessary to reach your goal. In other words, it can make your dreams and goals come true.

Extraordinarily successful people have been using this technique for ages. We all have this power within, but most have never been taught how to use it. It actually activates your creative subconscious mind, which provides you with ideas to take on and be successful in your journey.

It is a systematic process of mentally training your brain to think it has already achieved the goal, which you actually have not yet achieved. By visualizing it in steps -- over and over in your mind -- your brain over time believes it has already done the task, so, when you actually DO the task, you do it as if you've done it dozens of times already, which translates into you're easily accomplishing it.

Elite Olympic athletes use this method. A great example is 23-time Gold medalist Michael Phelps, who uses visualization. In his own words about visualization: "One of the things that has been good for me I think, besides training, has been my sort of mental preparation." 63

How it works is fascinating. Your brain has the ability to change "reality" through a process called neuroplasticity. By visualizing something over and over in your mind, it trains your brain to think it has already experienced that reality, which, actually, hasn't taken place.

I've been using visualization throughout my entire life, long before I even knew there was a name for what I was doing. It really works, and I highly recommend it to be used while adopting the plant-based diet. You can read more about it in my recent book *Becoming an Autism Success Story*.

In the beginning of my plant-based journey, I was visualizing that I could successfully make the transition to going plant-based by giving up ALL animal products. I had my eyes on the goal of reversing my diabetes and being totally in charge of my own health.

Chapter 11. Making Your Grocery List

This is a daunting area to discuss. I suggest you first make a list of the things you enjoy eating. Most things can be modified to fit a vegan dish. You will eventually learn to be creative. Between recipe books and the Internet, you won't lack for meal ideas. You can keep things really simple or you can learn to become a gourmet chef of plant-based cuisine! I am doing some of each.

I also recommend fun meals by taking aim at internationally-themed menus. I love Thai, Vietnamese, Mexican, all kinds of exotic delicious things I'd never had before until I found out about the whole food plant-based diet. Once you start thinking about *what* you want to eat, then you can begin planning your grocery list.

I would suggest keeping it simple in the beginning, so not to get discouraged. Now, I must make a confession. Well, maybe I shouldn't. In good conscience, I have no choice! My husband and I love to prepare and cook meals that are a bit more involved. Not every day, but most days. Due to our crazy, busy schedules, the pots, pans, skillets, dishes, bowls, forks, knives, and spoons end up piled everywhere in the kitchen! We use every last cooking utensil, which translates into everything being used up by Friday evening!

We never go out to eat, because everything is prepared at home. Yesterday was Friday. I looked around the kitchen and said to my husband, "So this is exactly what people will fear at the thought of going on the whole food plant-based diet!" We both burst out laughing!

While it is true that the kitchen gets very messy, the reward is that my diabetes has reversed, as has my high blood pressure, and I've lost 70 pounds so far. Abraham has lost 70 pounds also, and he feels the best he has ever felt.

If we kept up with the mess each day, it wouldn't get so out-of-control, but that's easier said than done! Life is full of choices. Our choice is to have great health and having fun doing it.

I'm going to give you a basic list to help you get started, but it is, by no means, the most comprehensive list out there.

Dark leafy greens are the most nutrient-dense of all foods. They are especially high in calcium, among numerous other nutrients. An interesting point to keep in mind is to "rotate" your greens. I recently attended an all-day workshop by Dr. Caldwell Esselstyn, one of the original pioneers of the whole food plant-based movement. During his presentation, he discussed the significance of eating dark greens every day, several times a day. Both he and his high-energy wife Ann want us to eat greens six times a day! Good grief! I know it!

Taking that a step further, he states it's important to eat all the different greens, not just one. For example, many people eat spinach greens every day. That's great, but each of the different greens has different vitamins, minerals and phytonutrients. By eating different ones each day, you are obtaining maximum health benefits.

I've got to tell you this! Both Dr. Esselstyn and his wife are like 87 years old, going on 40. They have been plant based for over 35 years, back when there were no computers to Google everything nor any cookbooks on this way of eating. Imagine starting out on such a huge endeavor? Dr. Esselstyn told me that his fellow physicians called him "Dr. Sprouts," his nickname for living the plant-based lifestyle and promoting it for his patients.

So that's what I mean by rotating your greens: eat all the different greens. You will be surprised at the vast difference in taste among each one. If you have a big salad every day, you can use that opportunity to incorporate several different kinds of greens, not only for the great variety of nutrition, but the different textures and tastes. You can squeeze the juice of a lemon or lime as your dressing or find an oil-free dressing recipe to use. In the last chapter, I provide several salad dressings to use on your greens or anything else. You can make up a batch and have it for a few days. They are not only delicious but pack a great nutrition punch too.

Here are some things to look for when shopping.

Fruits: Berries, lemons, limes, oranges, pears, peaches, bananas, cherries, mango, papaya, dragon fruit, cactus pear, apples. Pineapple and watermelon are ok too, in moderation. A note about grapefruit: grapefruit juice can affect numerous medications, which could lead to serious problems. If you plan to eat grapefruit or drink grapefruit juice, and you take any medications, you must refer to the following link for a complete list of drugs that can be affected by grapefruit and its juice. [14]

Vegetables: Basically, any vegetables available are great choices. I am sure I may have missed a few! Potatoes are fine as long as they are either Yukon Gold or sweet potatoes (orange or purple). Here you go. Asparagus, arugula, avocados, Bell Peppers, Bok Choy, Bean Sprouts, Beets (red and golden), Broccoli, Broccolini, Brussels Sprouts, Butternut Squash, Cabbage (red, green, Napa, purple), Carrots, Cauliflower, Celery, Chives, Corn, Daikon Radish, Cucumbers, Cilantro, Collards, Garlic, Ginger, Kale (green, red, Lacinto), Lemongrass, Mushrooms (cremini, oyster, portobello, shiitake), Mustard Greens, Onions (yellow, sweet, red), Parsnips, Parsley (Italian, curled leaf), Peas, Peppers (hot), Pumpkin, Radish, Rapini, Romaine Lettuce, Rutabagas, Spinach, Swiss Chard, Squash, Sweet Potatoes (orange and purple), Tomatoes, Turnips, Turnip Greens, Watercress,

Yams, Zucchini. See if your community has a farmer's market. You can usually find various produce there grown by local farmers, which will be literally just harvested.

Whole grains: Brown rice, rolled oats, corn, oat groats, winter wheatberries, faro, quinoa, barley, black rice, red rice, buckwheat, millet, bulgur, amaranth, spelt,

Legumes: Peas, chickpeas, lentils, black beans, cannellini beans, kidney beans, black beans, pinto beans, Navy beans, mung beans, split peas, red beans, black-eye peas, tofu, tempeh.

A note about tofu. The softer it is, the less fat it contains. For example, extra firm tofu has 6-7 grams of fat in a 4 oz. serving, while silken tofu has only 2 grams of fat. Neither has cholesterol. As you will learn about tofu and its use in recipes, the silken tofu is mainly used for making dressings, sauces, and smoothies. The extra-firm tofu is used for grilling, baking, sautéing and in soups and stews. It can be marinated and then cooked to your liking as the main course.

Unsweetened plant-based milks: Almond milk, soymilk. While oat milk is available, if you read the ingredients, it typically contains an oil as its second ingredient, so you want to avoid oat milk.

Herbs and Spices: Allspice, basil, black pepper, bay leaves, cardamom, chilies, cinnamon, curry, cloves, garlic, ginger, fennel, marjoram, mint leaves, nutmeg, dry mustard seed, paprika, rosemary, saffron, sage, thyme, turmeric.

All herbs and spices contain an abundance of protective phytochemicals and antioxidants, all of which are great for everyone, in particular, for those with diabetes.

There are numerous studies that show cinnamon helps in lowering blood sugar levels. I've seen similar articles on other things which may have similar effects, such as cayenne pepper, cloves, curry powder, garlic, ginger, marjoram, rosemary, sage. I personally use Ceylon cinnamon, as it has only trace amounts of coumarin, something toxic to the liver.

I like to buy fresh ginger root and turmeric, wash them, peel them, then thinly slice up some of each to toss into a pot of boiling water, then simmer for 10 minutes. You now have a delicious, nutritious tea loaded with anti-inflammatory and antioxidant power.

Spices are good for you and make food tasty and fun! Don't be afraid to try new tastes! Build yourself a collection of numerous spices. I like to arrange them in alphabetical order on a spice rack or in a drawer, so I can easily find what I'm looking for.

Herbs are a delicious and nutritious way to spruce up many recipes, salads, sandwiches, or spreads. Cilantro, parsley (regular and Flat Leaf Italian), basil, chives, dill, fennel, lemongrass, lavender, mint, sage, thyme. Each of these are highly fragrant and rich in flavor. Many are common to international cuisine but be adventuresome and incorporate these delightful and healthy items to any dish!

Condiments:

Salsa (sugar free and fat free), mustard, nutritional yeast, soy sauce, vinegar, lemon juice, lime juice. Always read the label to be sure they have no sugar or oil added. As time goes on, you will find many recipes to make your own dressings, salsas, and condiments that are oil free, sugar free, healthy and delicious.

Beverages

Coffee and tea with non-dairy unsweetened milk is OK. Water with a squeeze of fresh lime or lemon juice, and water, water, water, and more water!

Chapter 12. What Foods to Avoid and Minimize

OK. I've just got to say it! As I typed "Foods to Avoid or Minimize," it popped into my head to say, "pretty much everything you've *been* eating!"

The Whole Food Plant Based diet is a way of eating that focuses on consuming foods in their most natural form. This means that heavily processed foods are excluded. When purchasing groceries, focus on fresh foods, such as fruits, vegetables, whole grains, legumes.   When purchasing foods with a label, aim for items with the fewest possible ingredients. Most all of what I eat has just one ingredient. Apple. Broccoli. Cabbage. Onion. You get the picture. The longer the list of ingredients, the more highly processed it is, and the more bad things might be in there, which you don't want.

Foods to Avoid

- Avoid all animal products. I learned to not eat anything that has a mother or a face! This means no meat, chicken, pork, fish, eggs, milk, butter, yogurt, cheese, ice cream, sour cream, cream cheese, bone broth, collagen, casein (a milk protein), beef broth, chicken broth, candy (aside from high sugar content, many candies contain gelatin, which is obtained from the bones and skin of animals), chips (aside from the fact that they are from white potatoes and fried in oil -- depending on the flavor, some contain animal products such as whey, cheese or skim milk), Orange juice or any drinks that contain added Omega 3. This Omega 3 comes from fish oil or fish gelatin. Many salad dressings contain eggs, oils, and fish! It won't say fish on the ingredient list, but Worcestershire sauce, for example, contains anchovies! Some pastries are made with suet. Suet is the fatty tissue on the kidneys and loins of animals like cows and sheep.

- **Fast food:** French fries, cheeseburgers, hot dogs, chicken nuggets, or, basically, any fast food is food you want to pass by fast! Things like "healthy" subs are loaded with high fat lunch meats, carcinogenic preservatives, and even sugar added to the bread.

- **Added sugars and sweets:** Table sugar, soda, juice, pastries, cookies, candy, sweet tea, sugary cereals, lemonade, limeade, etc..

- **Refined grains:** White rice, white pasta, white bread, bagels, anything made with white flour.

- **Packaged and convenience foods:** Chips, crackers, cereal bars, protein bars, frozen dinners, etc. Start looking at the ingredient lists on packaged foods. It is usually a full paragraph loaded with nothing healthy, and even possibly carcinogenic.

- **Processed vegan-friendly foods:** Plant-based meats, faux cheeses, vegan butters, vegan mayonaise. Despite these foods don't contain any animal products, they contain oils and other unwanted ingredients. There are now many faux meats on the market, none of which I will eat.

- The closest I come to "alternative" burgers or hot dogs are burgers I make with mashed chickpeas, lentils, corn, bell peppers and spices that I grill and top with Romaine lettuce, red onions, tomatoes. For "hotdogs" I prepare carrots to use them instead, on a pumpernickel bun with chopped onions, stone ground mustard, and sauerkraut. I've served these burgers and hotdogs to friends who raved how delicious they were and demanded seconds! While these foods (processed vegan foods) can help you through the transition phase, I wouldn't recommend eating them on a regular basis.

I mentioned, they all contain a lot of oils, which you want to avoid or greatly minimize.

Artificial sweeteners Equal, Splenda, all of them. There are two reasons to ditch these items. First, you need to re-train your brain and palate (taste buds) not to crave sweet foods or drinks. Faster than you think, your cravings for sweet stuff rapidly changes, like within weeks. The second issue is that there is enough compelling research on the artificial sweeteners that they cause inflammation in the body. Inflammation is what you want to eliminate, as it causes a lot of damage and, even, is the basis for many diseases. These sweeteners also adversely affect the growth of "helpful gut bacteria." Beneficial bacteria are known to protect your gut against infection, produce important vitamins and nutrients, and even help regulate your immune system. So, the last thing you want to do is kill off the good bacteria! [15]

Chapter 13. What You Need to Prepare Your Kitchen

Kitchen tools

You will need a few things to make food preparation much easier. I don't want to overwhelm you by assembling a long list of equipment. There's also the cost factor for all these gadgets. I had pretty much all the tools you will eventually need, because I'm a gourmet chef and have been cooking my entire life since I was a young girl. Mom always had me by her side. From about age five, I'd be covered with flour as I was "helping" her. She taught me how to cook and bake from scratch. There are some real advantages to growing up poor! We couldn't afford to eat out or buy prepared food, so it all got cooked at home. At one point I was seriously thinking about a career as a professional chef. Now, I am putting my skills and knowledge to help others begin their own journey to great health.

Take inventory of what tools you already have available in your kitchen. Here are some of the most basic things you will need:

- Knives – Chef's knife and paring knife
- Knife sharpener
- Cutting board
- Measuring cup set
- Measuring spoon set

- Mixing bowls – various sizes
- Colander
- Nonstick skillet (I use Green Pan, a ceramic nonstick which is safer than Teflon)
- Saucepan – 3 quarts
- Soup pot, with lid – 12 quarts
- Soup ladle
- Can opener
- Garlic Press
- Food grater – handheld
- Silicone spatulas – various sizes
- Vegetable peeler
- Wooden spoons – 2
- Blender
- Food processor – I personally have the Ninja that comes with 4 attachments, including a 72 oz. blender, a 24 oz. Bullet blender, and food processor. It also comes with a blade that can make spiralized zucchini noodles. They are the workhorses of my kitchen.
- Steamer basket
- Rice Cooker – I see this as an essential piece of equipment because it allows you to cook not only rice (black, red, brown) but beans as well. Personally, I love to cook the dried beans of all kinds, as they have a much better, deeper flavor, plus no added salt or preservatives, which is what is in the canned beans. It

is also cheaper to buy dried beans in bulk.   You can purchase canned beans of all kinds – Chickpeas, Black beans, kidney beans, Navy beans, cannellini beans. I've never seen canned lentils or black-eyed peas, however. With a rice cooker, you don't need to soak beans overnight. You can simply add the dried beans to the rice cooker, add enough water to make it exactly one inch above the beans, place the cover on, and press the start button. In about forty-five minutes you will have delicious, perfect beans!

- Instant Pot - These include a rice cooker function and do so much more. You can sauté in it, even make non-dairy yogurt. They are all the rage!

- I like to use glass storage containers as they are the safest way to store food without worry of chemicals leaching into the food.

I need to talk a moment about knives and how to safely use them. Unless you are a seasoned cook and already know how to navigate your way in the kitchen, watch the video with this link[16]. https://www.youtube.com/watch?v=NlnOsnr94qM

Cookbooks I highly recommend investing in several plant-based cookbooks. My first suggestion is *Dr. Neal Barnard's Program* for *Reversing Diabetes Without Drugs,* which has numerous delicious and relatively simple recipes in it. His companion book *Cookbook for Reversing Diabetes* has 150 great recipes. I went the first few months using just these two books alone. I felt confident knowing that he approved each one, so I knew they were "diabetes safe." There are many other plant-based cookbooks, but you must get skilled to know what to omit, because the recipes might contain a lot of sugar. In those cases, you need to know what to replace the item with. You will need to be cautious of recipes even though they are plant- based, because not all plant-based recipes can be eaten by diabetics.

I recently attended an international plant-based conference at which breakfast, lunch, and dinner were provided. All plant-based but contained ingredients high in sugar. While the food was appropriate for most of the attendees, anyone with diabetes should not have eaten several of the items served. As time goes on, you will be interested to try new meals. You can also go online and find endless recipes and YouTube videos showing how to prepare the meals. Again, use caution with plant-based, evaluating each ingredient. If it says to use olive oil to sauté onions, you will use water or low-sodium vegetable broth to steam sauté your onions. It will become second nature on how to modify recipes to accommodate your special dietary needs.

I will explain how to steam sauté in just a bit! A plethora of great recipes is on the Physicians Committee for Responsible Medicine's site. Not only is it highly educational but click on the recipes' section for hundreds of great meals for breakfast, lunch, dinner, and snacks! www.pcrm.org

Chapter 14. Learning How to Read Food Labels

First, I must mention that manufacturers spend a lot of time and money designing their packaging. That is what first attracts the consumer to reach for that product. They do all kinds of things to entice you to buy the item, starting with labels that state, "Farm Fresh," "Gluten-Free," "All Natural." Because gluten allergies/intolerance is on the rise, you often see "Gluten Free" on labels of products that never even had gluten in them in the first place, like bagged limes with "Gluten Free" on the label. No lime has gluten, but they put it there to look more enticing.

Knowing exactly what is in a product is critical when purchasing food. On the whole food plant-based diet most of what you will be buying has only one ingredient, like apples, broccoli, or barley, for example. There will still be some things you will need that necessitate reading the label on the package. Canned beans, for example, typically only have beans, water, and salt, plus some kind of preservative. If you are not careful, however, there are some which may contain those ingredients *plus* pork or some other unwanted animal ingredient.

Even things like bread might contain eggs, butter, sugar, cane sugar, molasses, or some such thing. You can eat pumpernickel and rye. It's not only ingredients to be cautious of, however. It is serving size, servings per container, fat grams, sugar grams, sodium, and carbohydrates. Manufacturers are extremely talented in structuring their labels for consumers who do not read labels or don't know how to read the labels. The "serving size" stated on the label is a key factor, because the nutrition information might not seem so bad if you think the "serving size" is for the entire package or container. IF you read the label for further examination, there could be eight servings in total, so now you must multiply eight times each of the values to really know what is in the package.

For example, let's say it has 800 mg sodium in one serving. If you were planning to use the whole container, and there are eight servings, it now changes to 800 x 8 which is 6,400 mg of sodium. The American Heart Association recommends no more than 2,300 milligrams of sodium per day, and they are moving toward *an ideal limit of no more than 1,500 milligrams* sodium *per day*. As you can see, that container of food I'm using as an example contains 6,400 milligrams of sodium in total, which far exceeds what you should be ingesting. Even a seasoned shopper like myself is occasionally tricked by a label, not realizing something until I am home when I can take the time to further inspect the complete label and ingredients. When I say "tricked" I am referring to things like it will show zero sugar grams in the nutritional area. Yet, when reading the ingredients, cane sugar might be the fourth ingredient in the product. By law, manufacturers are not required to list things on the nutritional area if less than one gram. But it could be just a smidge under one gram and, to someone with diabetes, that might be enough to send their blood glucose way up.

As a person who will not eat any animal products, I've become even more aware of the significance of reading labels. I do not eat the "fake" meat products that are available nor any of the "fake" cheeses because there are lots of oils, like coconut oil, in the ingredients. Even worse, I noticed that one of the big companies who makes vegetarian breakfast items has the "fake" breakfast sausage links, which contain egg whites. For vegetarians who eat eggs and drink milk, it would be O.K., but for someone doing strict vegan, it's not O.K. When looking at the label to be sure there are no animal products, be aware that they might not be so obvious. Sure, if it says eggs, egg whites, egg yolks, milk or milk solids. That's easy to recognize. But you must also look for whey, gelatin, collagen, casein, sodium caseinate. These are all animal-derived products.

I cannot resist my temptation to tell you what gelatin is made from. It is made by prolonged boiling of skin, cartilage, and bones from animals. Basically, what's left over at the slaughterhouse: pork skins, horns, and cattle bones.

Collagen is equally as gross, made from cow hide, bones, or fish scales. I just read an article about a new diet craze that had me cringing for days. The diet has you using multiple scoops of collagen each day and sipping bone broth. Just the thought of all the cattle bones and connective tissue simmering away to make bone broth makes me sick.

If you need reading glasses to read small print, be sure to always carry a pair with you on shopping trips. That will save you time and money so you won't buy something that you thought was O.K. by glancing at the label, then getting it home to read the ingredients to discover something in it you don't want to ingest. Also, be very cautious with saturated fat! You want to steer clear of that, because as, you now know, it's fat that causes Type 2 Diabetes.

Read the ingredient list, which should be short and simple! I prefer my food to have one ingredient: apple. asparagus. cabbage. The more ingredients in a label, the more processed is the product. Manufacturers are required to list the ingredients in descending order by the amount used in the product.

Avoid products with white flour, wheat flour, enriched wheat flour, unbleached white flour, and fortified wheat flour.

Avoid oils. Yes, ALL oils. If you think olive oil is good for you, it isn't! Stay away from olive oil, canola oil, avocado oil, soybean oil, corn oil, vegetable oil, coconut oil, palm oil, sunflower oil, safflower oil, walnut oil, any oils. Also, avoid cocoa butter, butter, shortening (Crisco), lard (animal fat), any hydrogenated fats and oils, monoglycerides, diglycerides, and lecithin, which is a manufactured item made from soybean oil and, sometimes, egg yolks, none of which you want in your diet.

Watch out for sugar in any form. It might include multiple kinds of sugars. These include high-fructose corn syrup, dextrose, evaporated cane juice, cane juice extract, glucose, sucrose, honey, molasses, maltose, dextrose.

I'm going to mention **artificial sweeteners** again. I admit to having been hooked on several of them, namely Splenda and Equal. You can read dozens of articles about whether they are safe to consume, even if you don't have diabetes. An interesting thing I recently read was that the sight and smell of food, in addition to chewing and swallowing, triggers insulin to be released into your bloodstream. This is called "the cephalic phase insulin release," which translates into just looking at some food item which may be sweetened with artificial sweeteners can trigger an insulin response. I truly believe that if you want to be healthy, you must give up these chemically formulated sweeteners. You think you will never get over the cravings for those very things that brought you harm in the first place, but I can attest to the fact that your taste buds will change over time, and what you once thought tasted sweet and great will later taste terrible to you.

It is a gradual process, but it does really change. Artificial sweeteners also cause inflammation in the body, and, as I mentioned earlier, they affect gut bacteria.

Fats

This is an especially critical factor for those with diabetes. When purchasing any food product, be sure it has less than three grams of fat per serving. Where it shows "the percent of calories from fat," it must be below 10 percent. Remember, fat is what blocks insulin from entering cells to carry the glucose molecule inside; thus, the fat aggravates your insulin resistance. Indeed, your body does need a small amount of naturally occurring fat, which you can obtain from beans, vegetables, and fruits, which contain essential fats. These fats include alpha-linoleic acid and linoleic acid.

I'm sure you have seen all the hype about Burger King's new "Impossible Burger." The good news is that an animal didn't have to get slaughtered for it. The bad news is that it is high in fat: 34 grams, which contains saturated fat 11 grams; sodium 1080 mg; sugar 12 grams which equals three teaspoons of sugar. Plus, the patty is cooked on the same grill as the meat, so you would be getting the bacteria from the meat on your Impossible burger. There is a lawsuit filed against Burger King by a vegan regarding this very issue. I personally will not be tasting it, much less eating it. Dr. Neal Barnard's "take" on the Impossible Burger can be seen on a video[17]: https://www.youtube.com/watch?v=6ePOVdppS5s

Chapter 15. Meal Planning

I totally understand that you might feel overwhelmed wondering *what* to eat each day.

First, I'll tell you to take a deep breath and relax! With the plant-based movement gaining speed as it is, there's tons of meal planning ideas out there. There are even places around the country that make plant-based meals which are delivered right to your door. The one I'm most familiar with is Mama Sezz, as I've met the people who run it while at a conference in Oakland.[18]

I have learned to be very flexible and always be prepared. Let me explain what I mean. In the beginning I made up a calendar and planned out meals for each day. It seemed like a great way to be totally organized. But, then, I'd come home from work late, too tired to make what was on the calendar for that day. I'd feel guilty and upset that I wasn't following the plan. I came across a great article in the *Washingtonian*, on what Dr. Barnard eats in a day. I learned some great recipe ideas from it, but the biggest take-away for me was his plan for dinner each day of eating "beans, greens and grains." If you keep this rule of thumb in mind, you can easily assemble a healthy meal in no time flat. I have included the article in the footnotes[19]. You will enjoy it as much as I did, and it will give you a picture of the food too. Here is another thing you must see! Go on Dr. Barnard's www.pcrm.org website. In the "Search" area, type in "Power Plate". Wow. I'm salivating as I look at it. It will not only help you fully understand how you need to fill your plate, but he provides great recipes yet again!

The biggest tip I can give you on meal planning is to cook in bulk. When you have multiple food items stocked up on hand, you can quickly have a meal ready. Yes, you can plan ahead as much as you want. It is OK to eat the things you love on a regular basis. You must be sure, however, you are taking in enough of each category to be getting proper nutrients overall for each day. Take breakfast, for example. I tend to eat the same basic breakfast each morning with the exception that I occasionally fix something different on the weekends when there's more time.

However, I will cook up a huge pot of oat groats on Sunday to have ready to go for the next few days. Then at 3am on Monday morning, as I'm pouring my coffee, I can simply open the fridge and pull out that big pot (typically an eight quart Dutch oven pot) of oat groats, scoop out 1.5 cups into a big bowl, add some almond milk, heat it up and, then, add fruit. I love to cut up an apple, a banana, and berries, or papaya, kiwi, and Dragon fruit. There will always be two kinds of fruit in my bowl. I also add a teaspoon of Ceylon cinnamon, a tablespoon of freshly ground flaxseed, a tablespoon of ground hempseed, and a tablespoon of chia seeds. All that fruit? For someone with diabetes? Yes.

Back when I was going to that Primary Care Physician who told me to eat a Keto diet, there was no fruit of course, because he understood fruit contains sugar. As someone who loves fruit, I was devastated not being able to enjoy fresh fruit for nearly two years. Once I went plant-based I was able to start enjoying fruit every day. Lots of it. And I smile as I'm savoring each bite, thinking of that Primary Care Physician and his Google Glasses! Now I can eat that papaya like Dr. Nguyen was eating on that fateful phone call that led me to a plant-based lifestyle!

Because I am going to be eating oat groats and fruit for breakfast each day, that takes the stress out of breakfast.
I love to watch quick informative videos. Here is one of what Dr. Barnard and other top plant-based doctors eat in a day. [20]
https://www.youtube.com/watch?v=kjZUQb19fWg

Regarding lunch and dinner, once you have things cooked in bulk, that will enable you to have a variety of basics to get started to create a fun, healthy meal. In the last section of this book, I include a description of what I eat over a three-week period. There are recipes, but, perhaps, even more calming to you will be meal ideas. Instead of recipes that put many in a panic, I will explain how to use those bulk foods to create a delicious meal with minimal effort or thought.

Here is a fun fact! There is an acronym KISS, for "Keep it simple, stupid." This was started in the U.S. Navy in 1960 by an aircraft engineer, Kelly Johnson, the lead engineer at the Lockheed Skunk Works, which were the creators of the U-2 and SR-71 Blackbird spy planes. The KISS principle states that most systems work best if they are kept simple rather than made complicated; therefore, simplicity should be a key goal in design, so unnecessary complexity can be avoided. [21]

I have used the KISS principle throughout my entire life for so many things, to keep it simple. I utilize that same principle for the plant-based lifestyle! I have a very hectic schedule, as do most people. I'll help you get on track to stay there.

Chapter 16. Learning to Cook Without Oil or Butter

The most common question I get asked when people first learn about the plant-based lifestyle is "How can you cook without oil or butter?"   It's very simple. Instead, you'll use either water or low-sodium vegetable broth.

Here's all you need to do: Let's say you want to make New Orleans Red Beans and Rice. The recipe includes the "Holy Trinity" of green bell peppers, onions, and celery. Once you have these items chopped and diced, you sauté them until they are nearly caramelized. Using my green pan 12" skillet, I get it really hot. I do this by placing the pan on the stove burner and put the oven timer on for two minutes. That will get the skillet nice and hot. Once the timer goes off, you now toss in the chopped vegetables. They will make that enticing sizzling sound as they hit the skillet! Using two wooden, long-handled spoons, immediately begin stirring and gently tossing the veggies in the skillet. Continue doing this for several minutes. Have a small bowl sitting near you on the counter, with the water or broth in it and a tablespoon. That way it's right there to use as needed. When the vegetables look like they are beginning to stick to the bottom of the skillet, drop in one tablespoon of either water or the vegetable broth, whichever you are using. Of course, using vegetable broth will impart more flavor. When the liquid hits the skillet, it will send up a plume of hot steam, so be aware of this and do not have your face directly over the skillet.

Continue mixing and gently tossing the vegetables. Keep adding a tablespoon of the liquid as needed to keep the veggies from sticking to the pan and help them get caramelized. You will be pleasantly surprised at how nicely this method works, and how delicious the food will be. Be sure to scrape the browned patches in the skillet as you are adding each tablespoon of liquid. There's a lot of flavor there, and chefs always are sure to add those scrapings into the sauce or food to enhance the flavor. These are the little tricks I've learned over the years.

You will master it in no time. It just seems odd at first, but once you get the hang of it, you will feel like you have been doing it forever. You can practice sautéing the Holy Trinity!

Oh yes, here is my recipe for heart-heathy New Orleans Red Beans and Rice! I do a cooking class on the plant-based lifestyle at a local organic health food store each month. For the first class, I made this recipe which was a real hit, and everyone was eating second's and third's! I chose this recipe because down here in the South, Mardi Gras is a big deal, and I knew everyone would love it! Complete with zydeco music!

New Orleans Red Beans and Rice (Heart Healthy Version!)

Ingredient List

Table Salt

2-pound small red beans (about 4 cups) rinsed and checked for debris   Note: Camellia Brand red beans are best suited for this recipe, but not mandatory.

I medium yellow onion chopped fine (1 cup)

1 green Bell pepper – seeded and chopped fine (about ½ cup)

2 celery stalks – chopped fine (1/2 cup)

4 cloves garlic -peeled and minced (about 2 tablespoons)

1 teaspoon fresh thyme leaves

1 teaspoon smoked paprika

2 Bay leaves

½ teaspoon Cayenne pepper

½ teaspoon fresh ground black pepper

3 cups low sodium vegetable broth

6 cups water

2 teaspoons red wine vinegar, divided

2 tablespoons finely chopped fresh parsley

Brown Basmati rice – 4 cups cooked as you normally cook rice (I use a rice cooker, which has one rule of thumb: however much rice you put into rice cooker, add water to top out at one inch above the rice line.)

Hot sauce of choice

To prep the beans, you have two options:

1. **Overnight soak** – Into 4 quarts cold water stir in two tablespoons salt and two pounds of small red beans. Soak overnight at room temperature at least eight hours and up to 24 hours. Drain and rinse well.

or

2. **The "quick brine" method,** which is great as well. I use this method. Using a large Dutch oven, place 4 quarts water, 2 tablespoons salt, and 2 pounds small red beans. Bring to a boil over high heat. Remove the pot from the heat, cover, and let stand 1 hour. Drain and rinse the beans and proceed with the recipe.

In a large Dutch oven over medium-high heat, let the pot get nice and hot (I put the timer on for two minutes). If you haven't previously caramelized the onion, green pepper and celery, drop them in and begin stirring constantly. As previously stated, the vegetables will start to stick to bottom of pot. Toss in 1-2 tablespoon(s) low sodium vegetable broth and continue stirring. Continue stirring and adding water as needed to lightly brown the onions. They will begin to look caramelized, just as if you had used oil or butter. Once the onions are lightly browned and begin looking translucent, you are ready to proceed with the next step.

Stir in garlic, thyme, paprika, Bay leaves, cayenne pepper, black pepper, cook until fragrant, about 30 seconds. Stir in vegetable broth, water, and beans and bring to a boil over high heat. Reduce heat and vigorously simmer, stirring occasionally, until beans are just soft and liquid begins to thicken, which will be in about 45 to 60 minutes. Add 1 teaspoon red wine vinegar and stir well. Once the liquid has thickened, remove from heat, and add 1 teaspoon red wine vinegar and mix well again.

Ladle into bowls and top with a scoop of the Brown Basmati rice. Sprinkle the finely chopped parsley over the rice and beans. Serve with hot sauce of choice. Enjoy!

Cutting an Onion Without Crying!

Don't you just hate when you cut an onion and your eyes start burning and tearing? You just avoid cutting off the root end, which is where the gases are released that make you cry. The root end looks like strings coming out of the bottom, in case you don't know.

Chapter 17. How to Travel as Plant-Based Lifestyle

I travel a lot, flying to conferences, where I am speaking. Once I started on the plant-based lifestyle, I quickly realized you must do some planning ahead and be prepared to be creative. Despite the plant-based movement gaining rapid momentum, it's going to be difficult to find any venues at airports which serve food that will have plant-based menu options.

The first thing I learned to do is front-load my trip. What do I mean? Pack as many food items as you can for the initial trip to your destination. I typically fly everywhere. I cannot take liquids, but I can take a lot of things in separate bags packed in pockets and in carry-on luggage. I don't eat any nuts, because of the high fat content.

The day before departure, I'll bake up some tofu squares and pack them the next morning to carry with me. Be sure to refrigerate the tofu squares after cooking the day before, and pack them just before leaving the house for your trip. Typically, I will bring enough for the travel day. Be sure it's enough to eat but not too much that ends up having to get tossed the next day. I'll also cut up vegetables like cucumbers, carrots, bell peppers, to have those too. I love roasted chickpeas with spices on them. The day before, I will cook up a batch of chickpeas, toss them in my seven-spice blend, then roast them in the oven for 30 minutes. Once cooled they can be bagged up and stashed into every pocket and nook and cranny of your carry-on! The recipe for these is in the last chapter.

Find out ahead of time if the hotel you are staying at has a little refrigerator in the room or if you can have one brought to the room. Also go online and see if there are any grocery stores near the hotel. Then, you will know that, once you arrive at the hotel and get settled in, you can go get some fresh produce to continue your plant-based meals.

Some hotels have tiny kitchens or if you rent a cottage or house, which is becoming a trend, you might have a full kitchen to use. Then, you can cook while on your trip.

You can also search online for any vegan or Thai/Vietnamese restaurants nearby. These typically have vegetarian meal options. Mexican restaurants are also a good option to get plant-based food, like a bean burrito without cheese or sour cream. They do use oil to cook with, and they are usually accommodating if you tell them you are "deathly allergic" to oils! They know how to use water to spritz or to steam the vegetables.

At airports, your options will dwindle rapidly. At the biggest major airports across the country, there are chain restaurants, burger places, junk food and sugary drinks. You can look for restaurants that serve vegetables with their meals and ask to just get the vegetables, no oil, no butter, but that might be difficult for them. However, be prepared for some funny expressions from the person taking your order if you are in the United States. If you are in the UK, your chances of finding. plant-based meal options are greatly increased, as the plant-based movement is huge there. You won't get the funny looks when requesting special meal choices!

Also, when traveling, if you can find a local restaurant as opposed to a chain restaurant, you are more likely to have luck securing a plant-based meal. Often the local restaurants serve locally sourced produce, depending the location of the restaurant.

On the day of your departure from home, do plan to have a big, hearty breakfast. I will have my oat groats with berries, a banana, and an apple, plus a salad of greens like either fresh Swiss chard, collards, or red kale with a hint of balsamic vinegar drizzled over the greens. Then, I am set to go and won't be hungry anytime soon. Finally, stay active while on your trip. Whether you get out and walk for at least 30 minutes each day or work out in the hotel gym, get moving! I have never seen a hotel without a small (or large) exercise room that offers treadmills, weights, and, often, a pool too. Being on a trip or vacation doesn't mean you stop your normal routine.

Chapter 18. Eating Out

Of course, everyone enjoys going out with friends and family to eat out, celebrate birthdays, new jobs, achievements, or just because. Eating a plant-based diet doesn't mean you can't do those things any longer. It simply means you eat differently than before you went plant-based, but you still can go out and enjoy the company of friends and family.

One thing you will need to be prepared for is all the questions that you will be confronted with. Things like "why aren't you eating meat?" "How can you stand it not eating meat and cheese?" "I can't live without meat/cheese! How can you do it?" Remember that it is human nature to be so curious about something so significant like food. Always remember to be polite, and simply respond that you are doing it for your health. If they pursue questions about how will you get your protein, feel free to direct them to look at www.pcrm.org

Do not preach to others that they should be going plant-based. Hopefully, your success with it will be more than plenty for them to strike an interest in doing some research themselves. If they try offering you meat, cheese, anything like that, again, politely decline.

If you are invited as a guest to someone's home, ask if you may bring your favorite dish to share. That will serve two purposes!

First, you then know you will have at least one thing to eat! Second, others can sample your food and be pleasantly surprised, inspiring further constructive conversation about the plant-based lifestyle.

Chapter 19. Surviving the Holidays

I just went through my first Thanksgiving, Christmas, and New Year's Eve as plant-based. At first, in the days leading up to Thanksgiving, I was worried how it would affect me. It was the day before Thanksgiving, and I needed a few ingredients for our meal. My husband and I had discussed several times whether we wanted to make anything special for the holiday. Of course, it would be a plant-based dish, not deviating in any way, but perhaps something special. We decided upon a "comfort food" menu. As I wandered through the grocery store, I was very observant of other shoppers' carts and what food items were in them. Of course, everyone had all the traditional foods associated with Thanksgiving, turkey, ham, plus all kinds of cakes, pies, chips, junk food.

We had been going strong on a strict plant-based diet, which included no oils and no processed vegan foods such as vegan hotdogs, vegan cheese, vegan chicken. Nothing but fruits, vegetables, and whole grains and legumes. We still wanted to maintain our strict food but decided to make a few things which were labor intensive. The meal included mashed Yukon Gold potatoes smothered with a marsala-infused porcini-portobello mushroom reduction, chickpea and lentil loaf topped with a Ceylon cinnamon, apple, pear, dried unsweetened cranberry compote, corn cut off the cob, and vegan stuffing. We got adventuresome and even made vegan carrot cake cupcakes with icing made from raw cashews, dates, and Madagascar vanilla. We set up a small table in front of the fireplace with a lovely table setting and sat down to eat the feast. Only one thing was different. Neither one of us were too interested in eating the elaborate meal, least of all the cupcakes, despite how pretty they were. Oh, the food tasted great, but it was all too rich, and the cupcakes too sweet. A few bites of each item and we were done. Our taste buds had changed quite dramatically since May 13th when we first embarked on our plant-based lifestyle.

There was another compounding issue, I think. I always felt I never fit in anywhere because I am different from so many people. So now, I was the misfit who is plant-based and doesn't eat turkey to celebrate Thanksgiving. That thought made me feel even more alone and isolated than I typically felt. Then I realized something else. No turkey had to get killed for my dinner plate. That brought a sigh of relief to me and a feeling of inner peace. That made it all worth it. And then there was the reminder of why I'm doing this – to get rid of diabetes and get healthy. Done. End of feeling sorry for myself as a misfit. I felt a surge of pride in my accomplishment of going on and staying on the plant-based lifestyle. Christmas Eve and Christmas Day, we simply had our everyday fare. New Year's Eve was spent making Blue Corn Tortillas on our new cast iron tortilla press. We weren't making them because it was the holiday, only because the tortilla press had just arrived, and we were anxious to try it out.

There is one factor I did not have to deal with, and that's going out to holiday parties and family gatherings. Obviously, these events will be focused on food, food, and more food, most likely, none of which is going to fit into a plant-based diet.

I did a lot of research both on-line and by talking to seasoned vegans on how they handle the holiday family and friend gatherings. Here's what I learned. Eat before you go to an event. Offer the hostess to bring a vegan dish for others to try, then, you'll have at least one thing to eat!

Be prepared to be questioned by others about your new way of eating. Always answer them politely. Keep your answers positive. Don't start lecturing people about not eating meat.

Focus on the positive effects going vegan has had on your life. That will garner far more interest than preaching to others about what they're doing wrong.

Do not comment about the turkey. Chances are that you probably ate it at some point in your life. If anyone tries to coerce you into eating some, simply smile and say no thank you. Remember to truly celebrate the season. Yes, people will focus on the turkey, but there's plenty of other things to celebrate, like getting together with family and friends for a special memory-filled time.

There are plenty of festive foods to decorate the table at Thanksgiving and Christmas, from pumpkins, gourds, apples, squash, cranberries, oranges, cinnamon sticks, evergreen swags, poinsettias, holly, ornaments, candle-lit lanterns.

Yes, holidays are all about traditions, but there's no rulebook stating that new traditions can't be made! The most important thing is to smile, relax, enjoy visiting with those present, and have a great time.

Chapter 20.   Advice for Talking to Your Family and Friends

For those people closest to you, you might consider setting time aside to have a sit-down talk with them. It is human nature to resist significant changes, and that's what those around you see: a significant change.

If you have spent time with these individuals and went out for double bacon cheeseburgers together, they will immediately see that you can no longer share those same experiences. While switching to a plant-based diet has become much more mainstream recently, it can still be viewed as an "extreme" way of eating to many people. And when those people are your family and friends, it can be nerve-wracking to tell them you have gone plant-based.

The best thing to do is explain why you made this decision to go plant-based in a very matter-of-fact way. You can express that you would really appreciate it for them to support your decision. Explain that this is a new chapter in your life, a whole new lifestyle, and their support will mean the world to you. You can reassure them that you truly do understand that it seems weird, frustrating, and scary for them. State that there will be other ways to spend time together and connect.

Explain that just because you decided to make a change in what you eat doesn't mean that you have totally changed into a different person.

Well, I say this with some hesitation. Since becoming plant based, I have indeed changed very much as a person! All for the positive! Proceed to tell them you still like the things you normally do, but you decided to take your health into your own hands to make a positive change. Don't ever say anything to imply that they should go plant-based too. That is a personal decision for everyone. You were once in their shoes eating meat. You made this decision for your own personal reason. Think of the fact that you are planting a seed in their mind that might grow as time goes on.

Consider surprising them with some delicious plant-based food! Think of what you know they enjoy and make up a plant-based version of it. Perhaps, once they see how great it tastes, they won't be so freaked out. Remember the day I decided to go 100% plant-based and all that was left in my refrigerator was that head of broccoli? I think most people see this way of eating as all you can eat is some broccoli. Your job is to help them see that the sky's the limit with fabulous food that's plant-based.

I think an important thing at the conclusion of your conversation might be to ask them for their commitment to support you on your new journey. Keep it simple. And positive.

Hopefully, if they support you, they might ask questions about the plant-based diet, which will present teaching opportunities for you. Ultimately, always remember that you do not need their blessing to go plant-based. You know what is best for you and your health.

Chapter 21. Staying Motivated

For me, the biggest motivation was feeling better and better with each passing day! When you feel so sick for such a long time, each moment of gaining your health is the greatest gift of all. Also, to those you are closest too, whether it is a spouse, parent, children, friend, whoever. When they start seeing your health improve, it's going to make them happy too, which, in turn, will make you happy.

One thing that has happened to me since going plant-based is having thoughts of a particular food, but only when I see it. Let me explain. Let's say I'm at work and my boss orders 30 pizzas for all the anesthetists at lunchtime. There's a pizza place in town that makes these ginormous twenty-four-inch pizzas. In the past, I'd occasionally stop by there and get their Lunch Special, which was two HUGE slices of cheese pizza and a diet soda. I would sit at one of the tables by the window to eat my "treat." I'd block out everything, only to focus on the crispy, delicate crust, stretchy cheese, so hot it would burn the roof of my mouth. To counter that, I'd quickly take a sip of ice-cold diet soda. I was in 7th Heaven.

Oh yes, to make it all even worse, at each little bistro table they had multiple pizza toppings like grated parmesan cheese, oregano, and crushed red peppers. I would shake on some of each, especially the grated cheese to look like it was a grated parmesan slice. I'm cringing as I write about it. If I kept going like that, I'd really be in 7th Heaven. But here's what happens.

Just the other day, I walked into our lounge at lunch time. It was National Nurse Anesthetist Week, and each day we received a huge catered lunch from our boss. He always orders enough food to feed like 100 people, so there's food on every surface in the room! The moment I walked in, I saw huge pizza boxes stacked up everywhere, about 20 anesthetists eating those HUGE slices. Some were sprinkling on the grated parmesan, and the aroma all hit me like a TON of cinderblocks. No, not bricks. Cinderblocks. In that split-second moment of walking into all that, my mind felt a twinge of familiarity, of "normal." Like "oh, yeah! Sky's Pizza!" Then my conscious brain took over, and I walked right past the pizza, opened the refrigerator, and took out my lunch bag. I brought a huge wrap made from a giant collard leaf with numerous veggies, grilled tofu, and homemade hummus in it. I started eating, in my own little world. I focused on the crisp collard leaf that made a loud crunch sound each time I took a bite. I even had dipping sauce I made with silken tofu, garlic, cilantro, miso paste and lime juice. Several co-workers noticed my beautiful lunch and commented how delicious it looked. Never once did I feel sad that I wasn't eating the pizza. I felt incredibly empowered that I have the strength to stick with it no matter what.

Chapter 22. Learning to Cook in Bulk

Most people who follow the plant-based lifestyle learn to cook in bulk. This allows you to have numerous things on hand for the coming week. This cooking takes place on Sunday. It will all be used up by Thursday, but you can freeze food to have available for Friday.

This is where a big rice cooker comes in handy. Some things, however, are not suited for a rice cooker and must be made on the stove. An Instant Pot will work great too!

You can buy in bulk at many specialty stores that sell dried beans of all kinds, and many different grains. It is more cost effective to buy these items in bulk, especially the beans, and they are healthier too. Canned beans, while they are convenient, have added sodium and preservatives. Also, the dried beans you make at home in a rice cooker taste way better than canned beans. However, it's a good idea to always keep some canned beans on hand for those times when life gets in the way and you simply don't have the time to cook up a batch of beans! Trust me, I've been there and done that. In fact, because I live in Florida and need to be ready for hurricanes, my pantry is always stocked with about a dozen cans of each kind of bean. If I end up using some of them on those absolutely crazy days, the next time I'm shopping I just replenish them.

Here is what will get cooked on our Sundays (or whatever day you can be off from work to cook):

Black Rice – Cook in rice cooker / Instant Pot

Chickpeas – Rice cooker / Instant Pot

Quinoa – Cook on stovetop / Instant Pot

Winter Wheatberries – Stovetop

Barley – Stovetop

Buckwheat Groats - Stovetop

Oat Groats – These are whole oats. Totally unprocessed. I get a huge bag online from Amazon, a 15-pound bag of oat groats grown in Montana that looks like horse feed! These are the most nutritious oats on earth. They are organic and non-GMO. They must be cooked stovetop, however, in a big 8-quart Dutch oven pot. They take about 45 minutes to cook. What???? No eye-popping or jaw-dropping! Once you taste this oatmeal, you'll never want anything else. Aside from the delicious flavor, knowing how jam-packed full of nutrients and fiber they are will have you sold on them! Well, steel-cut oats are next best, followed by old-fashioned rolled oats.

Tofu

I like to either grill up or bake tofu slabs to have either as a snack, or with a meal. You will need extra firm tofu for this purpose. It is best to first squeeze out the excess water from the block of tofu. This can be done numerous ways.

Get a plate and place several thicknesses of paper towels on it, or a clean kitchen towel. Place the block of tofu on the plate and top with either more paper towels or kitchen towel. Place another plate on top of that, face down. Then pile some heavy books on top of the plate to weigh it down. Leave it all like that for at least 30 minutes. This will squeeze out the excess liquid in the tofu.

Another method is to use a special device made purposefully for this task, "a tofu tamer," as it's called. It is kind of like a vice which you place the tofu block between the two slabs and adjust the knobs to squeeze down, causing the same effect as the method described above. Leave this for at least 30 minutes just the same.

I hate to use this analogy, but it is the simplest way I can help you remember this. Think of tofu like chicken. If you don't marinate chicken or put some kind of herbs or rub on it, it's rather tasteless. The same holds true for tofu. On its own, it doesn't have a whole lot of flavor. But you can make tofu delicious with not much effort. Although I'm happy with it plain.

Ideas for marinades: Low sodium vegetable broth with some soy sauce, or teriyaki sauce, some freshly grated ginger, and some freshly minced garlic. This is a quick and easy way to go. Cut up your tofu after it's drained, place in a glass storage container and add the liquid. Place in fridge for 30 minutes.

Spices of your choice. I use my seven-spice mixture, added into some low sodium vegetable broth, or it can be used as a dry rub instead. Here's my mixture. It is one teaspoon of each item. You can place it all into a glass storage container and have it ready to go. Simply measure it all out then mix it all up. You don't need a lot, so then you will have the rest for other recipes.

- 1 tsp. Ancho Chili powder
- 1 tsp. Garlic powder
- 1 tsp Onion powder
- 1 tsp. Chili powder
- 1 tsp. Smoked Paprika
- 1 tsp. Cayenne
- 1 tsp. Chipotle Powder

You can either bake the tofu after its marinated or grill it up in a skillet using some low sodium vegetable broth just to wet the cooking process. Do not overcook the tofu. If using a skillet, just cook on medium to medium-high, several minutes on each side until lightly browned. To bake it, I set the oven at 325 degrees and bake 20-30 minutes. Depending on your desired taste, you might want to turn them over and bake another 12-15 minutes if you want the tofu crispy. After its cooled, store any unused tofu in a glass storage container up to two days. I take several pieces each day to work as my mid-morning snack, along with a half cup black rice.

Soups – If you have the time, cooking up a nice big pot of a hearty soup is a great dinner option for a few dinners, and you can always freeze some to have on hand for those days you need a really quick option! Check out the last chapter here in this book for some great soup ideas. There you will find my Miso Soup recipe, and Black Bean Soup.

When you have all or most of these items ready to go, you can put together a healthy, satisfying meal in no time flat. Remember that saying by Dr. Neal Barnard, "beans, greens, and grains." You can take a few pieces of tofu, some black rice, bake a sweet potato, and rustle up a side salad of greens! Voila!

Snacks -- Everyone loves to snack on something! For me I love to eat things that crunch! There are tons of things you can have as a snack, not just carrot sticks! Be creative! Think outside the box. One of my favorite snacks is air popped organic popcorn with nutritional yeast sprinkled all over it. Or baked chickpeas with my 7-spice blend sprinkled over it. Or about 1 tablespoon blue agave syrup mixed into 4 tablespoons water, put into a tiny spray bottle, and spritz over the popped corn and bake on a cookie sheet for 12 minutes. You can purchase a tiny spray bottle intended for food purposes.

You can make hummus with chickpeas and lemon juice to use as a dip or spread on a collard leaf and roll it up.

I just discovered that when eating an apple, if I sprinkle on a very faint touch of salt, it takes the flavor to a whole new level. Use the salt extremely sparingly. Wow.

Check out the last chapter of the book for recipe ideas. I'll bet you are just like me, looking for recipes that are quick and easy yet healthy and nutritious. When you get a case of the munchies, you will be prepared.

Chapter 23. Food Safety

I am the world's biggest advocate for food safety, probably to the point of being ridiculous. I rarely eat out, even before going plant-based. Unless I could see that the people handling the food wear gloves, I would not eat there.

Many years ago, when I lived up in Pennsylvania, I got food poisoning so bad I had to be hospitalized. I will never forget that experience. Dozens of people who ate at that restaurant also got sick. It all was from a food handler, who contaminated everything with his filthy hands. Even before that event I was a big fan of ultra clean handling of food. After that I was even more stringent.

Here is some data that will help you understand my obsession for food safety. The CDC estimates that each year **48 million people** get sick from a foodborne illness; **128,000** are hospitalized; and **3,000** die. As a healthcare provider, I look at those numbers and want to cry. It is mostly preventable. 22

A report from the World Health Organization published Dec. 3, 2019, is the first to estimate the worldwide burden of foodborne illnesses. The numbers we had before were not comprehensive or global.

One of the most disturbing findings from the report is that children are disproportionately affected: 125,000 kids under five die from foodborne illnesses every year.[23]

"Based on what we know now, it is apparent that the global burden of foodborne diseases is considerable, affecting people all over the world — particularly children under five years of age and people in low-income areas," Dr. Kazuaki Miyagishima, the WHO's Director of Food Safety and Zoonoses, said in the agency's press release.

The biggest causes of foodborne illness are diarrheal diseases like norovirus, Campylobacter, Salmonella, and E. coli, according to the report.[24]

Campylobacter can be found on almost half of the chicken sold in grocery stores, and Salmonella and E. coli are found on raw meat as well as elsewhere. In many cases, the illness can be prevented by simply cooking meat properly, which means that raw meat must be handled carefully, and cooking meat should be cooked all the way through. Meat is not always the culprit: a recent E. coli outbreak in the US was traced to celery.

Norovirus, which often makes headlines when it causes outbreaks on cruise ships, can be transferred to any food that infected people touch, if they don't wash their hands properly.

There are more than 250 different foodborne diseases, which are caused by bacteria, viruses, and parasites. E. coli, for example, is a bacterium, while Hepatitis A is a virus, and Taenia solium is a tapeworm parasite found in pork. [22]

Fortunately, when you go plant-based, you have just significantly decreased the deadly bacteria coming into your home, because you are not bringing in any meat, chicken, pork, or eggs. I frequently see news reports of millions of pounds of meat or chicken recalled, because it is contaminated with salmonella or E. coli.

Unfortunately, that's not to say vegetables or fruits can't be contaminated with such microorganisms. You must do your part not to contaminate them as well, when you are handling food.

Whew! I don't have to talk about handling raw meat, pork, or chicken! That's quite a long topic.

Let's talk about what does concern you on your plant-based lifestyle. The first thing you need to do before any food preparation is thoroughly wash your hands, preferably with antibacterial hand soap. If you are going to be preparing food for others, you need to wear food handlers' gloves, to be donned AFTER you wash your hands. As you go along in your preparation, wash your hands again if you handle anything considered contaminated.

I highly recommend you invest in a salad spinner if you don't already have one. They are relatively inexpensive. You will be eating a lot of greens, and you must wash them all prior to consuming. Everything must be washed: Cilantro, parsley, things that might just be used as decorative or a garnish, as well. That bunch of cilantro might be contaminated from the soil it grew in, or contaminated water used to grow it, or unsanitary workers who are harvesting it, or by multiple hands by workers packing it to be shipped, or those at the grocery store who put on display, and, even more, as customers handle bunches looking for their favorite one. That seemingly innocent little bunch of cilantro could be infested with E. coli, salmonella, Listeria, even Hepatitis A. Wow.

Sorry to be the messenger. There have been numerous food poisoning cases from fruits and vegetables, especially because these items are typically eaten raw. To minimize your risk, always wash your greens thoroughly before eating.

I get a large bowl and fill it with cool water, and I add a few drops of antibacterial dish detergent. The FDA does not recommend using any type of soap, because it might not be thoroughly rinsed off, and soap is not intended to be consumed. I will admit to finding that a contradiction, because food products like fruits and vegetables are sprayed with toxic chemicals for pesticides and herbicides. You cannot always find organic items, and some people simply can't afford to buy organic. With that said, I always thoroughly rinse each leaf. I can taste the soap if it isn't all rinsed off. When I think of all the possible bacteria that could be present on the greens, that outweighs the risk of the soap for me. You do not have to do what I do, but I want to say exactly how I clean my greens, fruits and vegetables.

After filling the bowl with the cool water and a few drops of dish detergent, I get the greens -- say a bunch of mustard greens -- and cut off the end of it. Examine the leaves for any brown or damaged areas and remove those. Submerge all the now loose leaves under the water and very gently swish back and forth. Leaf by leaf, I pick out, gently wash with my hands, then very thoroughly rinse until squeaky clean. Then, I place it into the salad spinner. Once the spinner is full, place the lid on it and lock down, then spin the handle being careful not to get your fingers caught in the open area on top. I suggest reading the instructions which come with the salad spinner prior to using. Now, your greens are clean, dry, and ready to use.

Rice is another thing you will probably be eating a lot of. Black, red, brown. Your choice. Surprisingly, rice is a high-risk food when it comes to food poisoning. Uncooked rice can be contaminated with spores of a *bacillus cereus* bacterium that produces toxins that cause food poisoning. These spores can live in dry conditions. For example, they can survive in a package of uncooked rice in your pantry. They can also survive the cooking process. If cooked rice is left standing at room temperature, these spores grow into bacteria that thrive and multiply in the warm, moist environment. The longer rice is left standing at room temperature, the more likely it will be unsafe to eat. To reduce your risk, serve the rice as soon as it has been cooked and refrigerate leftover rice as quickly as possible after cooking. When reheating cooked rice, make sure it is steaming hot all the way through. [25]

A number of fruits – namely, berries and melons -- have been linked to food poisoning outbreaks. Fruits such as cantaloupe, honeydew, and watermelon can be contaminated with Listeria, which grows on the rind then infiltrates into the flesh. Between 1973 and 2011, there were 34 reported outbreaks of food poisoning associated with melons in the US. This resulted in 3,602 reported cases of illness, 322 hospitalizations and 46 deaths.

Cantaloupes accounted for 56% of the outbreaks, watermelons accounted for 38% and honeydew melons accounted for 6%. Fresh and frozen berries, including raspberries, blackberries, strawberries, and blueberries, are also a common source of food poisoning due to harmful viruses and bacteria, particularly the hepatitis A virus.

The main causes of berry contamination include being grown in contaminated water, poor hygiene practices of berry pickers, and cross-contamination with infected berries during processing. [24]

Raw sprouts, including alfalfa, mung bean and clover sprouts are common sources of salmonella, *E. coli*, and Listeria. Sprouts grow in moist, warm conditions and are an ideal environment for the growth of bacteria. Cooking sprouts can help reduce the risk of food poisoning. [25]

I love bean sprouts from mung beans and grow them at home. It's quite easy to do, and, at least, I can control the conditions they are grown under.

I don't mean to scare you, but, instead, make you aware of dangers lurking right in your home that you can address by proper food handling, cleaning, and cooking practices. It might also inspire you to start your own garden, even if it's just herbs in containers on your windowsill or, if you have the interest and space, you might like to get into raised bed gardening or tiered gardening. Not only could you then control what goes into the plants, it's relaxing, and you can get your vitamin D3 while tending your garden in the sunshine!

Be sure to thoroughly wash each fruit and vegetable before preparing the meal. I love washing bell peppers, as I love that squeaking sound they make as you are rinsing them! Cucumbers, of course, need to be very thoroughly washed.

Another rule of thumb. Date everything you put into storage containers. You do not want to "wing it," as you ponder just how many days ago you cooked it. If there's no place to write the date, simply get a sticky note pad and write the date on it and stick it onto the glass container. The safest choice for food storage is glass containers.

Chapter 24. Necessary Supplements

Vitamin B 12 - Vitamin B12 is naturally found in animal products, including fish, meat, poultry, eggs, milk, and milk products. Vitamin B12 is generally not present in plant foods. For this reason, when you are on a plant-based lifestyle, you need to take Vitamin B12 supplements, which provide a minimum of five micrograms per day. According to Dr. Barnard, "many people, particularly older people, tend to run low on vitamin B12 regardless of their diets, because their bodies become less efficient absorbing it. That is also true of people taking metformin or acid-blocking medications." *Dr. Neal Barnard's Program for Reversing Diabetes Without Drugs,* pg.144.

Vitamin B12 is required for proper red blood cell formation, neurological function, and DNA synthesis.

In addition to vitamin B12 supplements, nutritional yeast is another good source of B12, which can be added to recipes, sprinkled over vegetables, and even used to make "nacho cheese sauce!" It has a nutty cheese-like flavor. Again, you will need to read the label to determine the serving size and vitamin B12 content.

I feel compelled to include this information. There have been recent studies like this one in Journal of the American Medical Association (JAMA) Network. Their study about vitamin B-12 says "These findings suggest that higher levels of plasma concentrations of vitamin B_{12} were associated with increased risk of all-cause mortality after adjusting for age, sex, renal function, and other clinical and laboratory variables. The mechanisms underlying this association remain to be established." [26]

For this reason, I personally only take a B-12 supplement once a week, and it is the lowest dose, which Dr. Barnard talks about. If I make recipes that include the nutritional yeast which contains B-12, I omit my supplement that week. That is my personal approach. Check with your doctor on whether you should be taking B-12 for your needs. You can also get a blood test to determine your B-12 level.

Vitamin D

Vitamin D3 is a fat-soluble vitamin that helps your body absorb calcium and phosphorus. Having the right amount of vitamin D3, calcium, and phosphorus is important for building and keeping strong bones. Vitamin D is used to treat and D3 prevents bone disorders. Vitamin D is also made by the body when skin is exposed to sunlight. However, protective clothing, sunscreen, limited exposure to sunlight, dark skin, and age may prevent you from getting enough vitamin D from the sun. Unfortunately, over 75% of the US population is vitamin D deficient. Vitamin D helps regulate your entire immune and neuromuscular system, helping reduce inflammation throughout your muscles and joints, and it fights off infection. It is easy for the government to track vitamin D deficiencies of the population. Each day as I read through patients' Electronic Medical Records, I see vitamin D deficiency in at least 75% of them. All that data is reported to the government. Young and old, it is a pretty common issue.

There are several points I'd like to make. It is true that regular sun exposure is the best way to get vitamin D. Twenty minutes several times per week will do it. Factors to consider are your skin color (darker skin may need a little more than 20 minutes); how far you live from the equator (the farther away from the equator, the more sunlight you'll need); how much skin you expose to the sunlight; and whether you are wearing sunscreen. Important: after that 20-minute exposure, apply your sunscreen to help prevent skin cancer!

One last thing. I discovered that vitamin D3 supplements

typically found in drugstores, supermarkets, etc. are manufactured from sheep grease. Yup, the lanolin is derived from their wool, which is skimmed off the water after they boil the wool. It is a yellow waxy substance that makes the sheep "waterproof." There is an alternative, thankfully! There is a plant-based source made from lichen and can be found on-line or in specialty food stores as Vegan D3.

Here is a fun fact! Vitamin D2 can be obtained by eating mushrooms which have been exposed to natural sunlight, which increases their Vitamin D2 content. You can do this yourself by getting shiitake mushrooms, removing the stems, and placing them gill-side up in direct sunlight from 10am to 4 pm for two days. You then dry them and place them in a glass storage jar. If you slice the caps and spread them out for their sunbathing time, they will produce even more Vitamin D2. Studies show no real difference in this D2 compared with supplemental D3 taken in pill form. Moreover, eating mushrooms packed with vitamin D2 confers many other health benefits because mushrooms have many helpful nutrients, including beta glucans for immune enhancement, ergothioneines for antioxidative potentiation, nerve growth stimulators for helping brain function, and antimicrobial compounds for limiting viruses.

You might be envisioning me outside on a bright sunny morning spreading out several pounds of sliced shiitake mushrooms to catch some rays. Indeed, you are correct! I have read about twenty supporting articles backing this information. Here is the article I obtained the above data from. I highly suggest reading it!.[27]

Chapter 25. A Word About Exercise

That dreaded word. Here's what I'll share with you. When I started the plant-based lifestyle, I was too sick to think about exercising. I literally felt like I was on the verge of dying. Each step to get into the hospital each morning for work was an ordeal. I was gasping for breath, wondering how much longer my body could go on like this.

Now, I use that long distance to do my powerwalking to perk myself up. I work out at home after work, six days a week. Very rapidly, like within a few weeks, I began feeling a whole lot better and started having energy. I then wanted to move, walk, and work out. Exercise is good for everyone, but, in particular, it is critical for those with diabetes. As always, talk to your doctor before starting any exercise or new way of eating to be sure it's right for you.

Walking is the simplest, least intimidating exercise that most people can do. Start out slowly. Try to walk 30 minutes five days a week. If you can only walk two minutes in the beginning, do not fret. Just do what you can safely do. And do not get sad or feel like "what's the point?" The point is that each step you take is another step in the right direction. Have you ever heard the saying, "Rome wasn't built in a day"? It is an adage attesting to the need for time to create great things! It is the usual English translation of a medieval French phrase. It took many years to get where you are at right now. It will take time to get your health under control, but learn to have **Patience**, **Perseverance**, and **Positive thinking**! The three P's!

Chapter 26. Talking to Your Doctor About Going Plant-Based

This is not going to be an easy task! If you happen to live in the Washington, D.C. area and end up at the Bernard Medical Center, you are in luck!

But, most of us are going to be dealing with physicians just like that one who fired me from his practice. They have zero knowledge of nutrition and, least of all, the power of the plant-based diet. Keep in mind, you cannot hold this against them. Until only recently, medical schools had provided little, if any, education in this area. Thus, physicians are out there prescribing billions of dollars of pills, procedures, and surgery. That is the way they were taught, so that's what you get.

Here is another issue to toss out there. Most doctors do not like being told by their patients what the patient wants to do. The doctors are used to being in charge and telling you what to do, and they believe they know best. They are not used to having a patient who wants to take their health into their own hands. I do not doubt that there is a possibility that you might get fired by your physician when you tell them you want to (or already have) gone plant-based. It is going to depend on how you present it to them. Doing so in a non-confrontational style will create the best results.

On my website is a superb video of my interview with Dr. Neal Barnard, as he talks about this very topic. I highly recommend you watch it at www.yourwfpblife.com

You do need to keep up your end of this deal. Stick with the plant-based eating. Write down what you eat, so you can show your doctor.

You must check your blood sugar very frequently, at least for the first few months. I was checking mine when I first got up in the morning, after I ate breakfast, mid-morning, before/after lunch, when I got home, before/after exercising, before bedtime. Ouch. No kidding. My fingertips were sore after all that, but I needed to know what was going on. Write it down. Your doctor will be pleased that you are so diligent. They will also be curious as to what really is going on after you start the plant-based diet. This will, most likely, all be new to them. When I started my plant-based diet, my A1C was 12.4. It is now 5.9! Know all your numbers! Be prepared to be met with resistance. It might go something like this:

"I've been struggling so long with my Type 2 Diabetes, and all the medications, insulin, side effects, I simply wanting to improve my health. I've discovered that the plant-based diet can prevent, treat, and even reverse diabetes! It's all backed by research. I have read all about it and I want to go on it. I am going to need your help, by regulating my medications, which will need to be decreased, possibly even discontinued over time. I really want to be as healthy as possible, and I'm committed to stick with this plan."

At that point, you can show him/her something like Dr. Barnard's book *Reversing Diabetes Without Drugs* or even something like the *For Your Doctor Kit* from pcrm.org[28] This is information specifically for physicians and health care providers.

You can tell them about the thousands of success stories you have heard or read about, and you'd like to be another success story. Once the doctor sees that you are committed, serious, and even have literature to back it up, she/he hopefully will take it as a learning opportunity. If, however, they do not accept this and they fire you, just smile and look for a plant-based physician who will embrace your decision. Telemedicine and Telehealth are popular sites, so they might enable you to find a plant-based doctor best suited for you.

Telemedicine involves the use of electronic communications and software to provide clinical services to patients without an in-person visit. Telemedicine technology is frequently used for follow-up visits, management of chronic conditions, medication management, specialist consultation and a host of other clinical services that can be provided remotely via secure video and audio connections.

The term "telehealth" includes a broad range of technologies and services to provide patient care and improve the healthcare delivery system. Telehealth is different from telemedicine, because it refers to a broader scope of remote healthcare services than telemedicine. While telemedicine refers specifically to remote clinical services, telehealth can refer to remote non-clinical services, such as provider training, administrative meetings, and continuing medical education, in addition to clinical services. According to the World Health Organization, telehealth includes, "Surveillance, health promotion and public health functions." [29]

Eventually, there could come a time, when it will be mainstream for physicians to offer each patient the choice of choosing the plant-based diet as the first line of choice to treat their ailment. There are many things being done by the pioneering physicians out there on the front lines fighting for the plant-based movement to prevail. These range from mandatory Continuing Medical Education to bills passed in states requiring every hospital to offer plant-based meal options to patients and even insurance companies recognizing the power of plant-based by reimbursing physicians for related activities. It is going to win.

Dr. Barnard is at the tip of the spear of all this. You are now part of this momentum! Do you realize that planting a seed in your doctor's mind will hopefully grow, leading him/her to understand this need, and offering it to all his/her patients?

Each little piece of the puzzle eventually leads to completing the big picture. Each step that every person takes is opening more doors to better health for everyone.

Let the journey begin, one meal at a time!

Part 3:
For Physicians

Chapter 27. For Physicians Only - It Is What It Is

The whole food plant-based diet is gaining speed by the day. The momentum is here, and its coming like a tsunami. It is not just for good health but, also, for preventing, treating, and reversing many chronic and inflammatory diseases. It is also an excellent, safe, and healthy way for your obese patients to lose weight.

As a physician, you have an opportunity to make a significant impact with your patients. You cannot ignore facts. You cannot ignore reality. It is time to take a serious look at this and adjust the way you do your job as a physician. There are significant research-proven results to solidify the power of a plant-based diet. There are now thousands of individuals with a success story that proves beyond a doubt that this really works. There are answers that are not in the pharmaceutical world, and they are proven answers. Until you address this, you are doing a disservice to your patients.

Don't assume that patients won't have the motivation to go on this lifestyle. You will be very surprised how many *will* go on it and *stay* on it. But they must be given this option as a way of treating their disease(s). Once they see how quickly they begin to feel better and feel empowered by taking control of their health, that will be the impetus they need to continue the journey. From the healthcare dollars' standpoint, physicians need to realize the effects of healthy food choices on reducing the costs of healthcare. I realize that physicians are trained to treat the symptoms of diseases rather than address the disease itself, but this must change.

Most physicians receive little, if any, education on nutrition in medical school or residency. You will need to take the initiave and begin learning about the power of a whole food plant-based diet to start thinking about how to get your patients moving in this direction.

Once a patient adopts this lifestyle, you will need to begin evaluating their changing needs and have their medications readjusted, and, at some point, possibly discontinue the medications altogether. In the world of Type 2 Diabetes, this is a foreign concept to most physicians, because the normal route is to increase patients' medications and dosages.

With a whole food plant-based diet, changes will start happening rather quickly, generally within the first two weeks and continue improving as time goes on. Particularly important is working with the diabetic patients on insulin and glucose lowering drugs. These patients typically know how to deal with the high BG levels, but their BG will start dropping dramatically, so they need to be careful of not "overdoing it" with regular dosages of their insulin and other medications. They will have to check their BG numbers more frequently to know how they are progressing, especially at nighttime, when their BG might be dropping far below what they normally had prior to going on the plant-based diet.

Obviously, this will require consultation with each patient in the initial phase. A helpful reference is the short video on my website www.yourwfpblife.com by Dr. Neal Barnard, who explains how he handles the patients' transition at his medical center.

Points to consider are the disease process of diabetes and the role fats play in insulin resistance. Perhaps a drawing can be made for the patient to show how fats block the receptor sites on the cells, which prevent the insulin from carrying the glucose molecule inside the cell. Seeing a visual rendition will help the patient understand what's really going on. Patients are likely to pay attention positively to the impacts of the following: the reduction of using insulin, which is inconvenient at the least; the elimination of the costs of their diabetes' medications; and the savings in their budget, once they learn how to batch cook and how to eat this way.

A big hurdle for many people is to change what they order when going out to eat. You might have to work with the whole family, to explain this program and, hopefully, get them on board. Even their children. Milk is another problem. You need to learn about the dangers to everyone's health from drinking milk. Yes, you are used to believing that milk and milk products are healthy, and children and teens need to drink it for proper growth and development. There are strong supporting studies that show quite the opposite, of the negative and very unhealthy effects milk has on the human body. Here is one of many supporting articles about milk and the protein casein.[30] Wow. I know. This is a lot to hit you with.

There is a great documentary (on YouTube) that I highly suggest you see, to learn the influences the big industries have on marketing the very products that are making hundreds of millions sicker every day. Here is an eye-opening documentary everyone needs to see. [31]

It might take some time to change your focus from writing out prescriptions to enabling the patient to take charge of their own health. But once you know the facts, it will be easier.

I am reaching out to you as both a fellow healthcare provider but, mostly, as a patient. I know you are busy, so I will keep this brief. When I discovered I have Type 2 Diabetes, my

Primary Care Physician lacked any knowledge of the whole food plant-based diet. The only avenue of treatment he was familiar with was to reach for his prescription pad to start writing out the usual drill: Metformin; Sulfonylureas, such as glipizide; DPP-4 inhibitors such as Januvia; GLP-1 receptor agonists such as Victoza; and insulin. In my case, any or all these drugs caused side effects, which can range from mild to unpleasant, to life-threatening and, even, death.

While it is true that most patients take these pills everyday with few side effects, there are some who aren't so lucky. Some patients, like myself, are super sensitive to most all drugs and are unable to take them. It is also becoming more prevalent that individuals seek to find a natural way to address their health issues because of that. Even more, by handing out prescriptions for Type 2 Diabetes, you are treating the symptoms, *not* the problem itself.

Take diabetes, for example. The various drugs do a number of things, including reducing the absorption of glucose, reducing the release of glycogen, while another class of drugs increases the body's sensitivity to insulin. Another drug acts to kickstart the pancreas' release of more insulin. Another increases insulin production in the pancreas and decreases glycogen, while yet another blocks glucose from being absorbed into the kidneys and causes it to be eliminated through the urine instead. Often, patients are given several different drugs as each one does different things. They all come with a cost, not simply monetarily, but with the side effects which come along with them. Speaking of cost, many patients with diabetes or any other conditions are elderly on fixed incomes, often near poverty level. Many of these prescriptions are very expensive and can mean the difference of them not having money for food or heat in order to purchase their pills.

The whole food plant-based diet will clean out the intramyocellular lipids to allow insulin to transport the glucose molecules inside the cells where they belong. Not only will the patient's blood glucose levels drop, their energy level will dramatically increase. Additionally, there are no Black Box Warnings on the whole food plant-based diet.

The side effects of the whole food plant-based diet are dramatically improved health, and reversing diabetes, heart disease, weight loss, and more.

That's a win-win situation. This diet will enable the patient's body to begin functioning normally. Isn't that the optimal goal? Not to simply mask the problem but address the actual cause and fight the disease? Hopefully, once you incorporate the plant-based diet as a consideration into your practice, you will reach for a shopping list in the produce aisle instead of reaching for your prescription pad.

As a healthcare provider, I also know that most physicians see medications as their first and *only* line of defence against diseases. Over my thirty-plus year career as a Certified Registered Nurse Anesthetist, I've seen firsthand the lure of big pharmaceutical companies on anesthesia providers. Huge, expensive catered lunches in the lounges and the fancy dinners at the most expensive restaurants in town so they can eat and listen to the guest speaker the pharmaceutical company has flown in to talk about their drugs for us to use. The same goes on for every branch of medicine impacted by these huge corporations. I am happy to see that this trend is changing, and drug reps are no longer luring healthcare providers with expensive meals, at least in some health care facilities. The hospital where I work no longer allows this to go on. That is great news. Hopefully, every institution across America will adopt this standard.

However, the marketing doesn't stop with the healthcare providers. The TV networks are laced with advertisements by pharmaceutical companies, seeking to influence the consumers (patients) with the diseases like diabetes, heart disease, inflammatory diseases, even cancer. I will hear the ad talking up the new drug, like it's the greatest thing since sliced bread, and, yes, they will even mention all the possible deleterious side effects and even death. They say it so softly and pleasantly that it makes it sound OK if you get acute liver failure and die.

In today's information age, more and more people are turning to the Internet to seek answers about their health issues and alternative treatments. That is exactly what I did, for nearly two years. Yet, never in my searches for a cure or alternative way to treat Type 2 Diabetes did I come across *anything* about Dr. Neal Barnard nor the whole food plant-based diet as a way to address it. Why didn't my Primary Care Physician know about this? Despite my literally begging him for a natural way to treat my diabetes, he was not informed in medical school or the literature subsequently, so he told me there wasn't any alternative. He simply continued to write the scripts for the products produced by BIG Pharma.

The whole food plant-based diet is not just for reversing diabetes. It can reverse heart disease, inflammatory diseases, and, even, some cancers, according to evidence-backed research.

It is a sad fact that nutrition is addressed little -- if any -- in medical school. As a result, you possibly and other physicians out there on the front lines are unaware of the power of the plant-based diet. Thankfully, this is beginning to change, with the work of pioneering physicians like Dr. Neal Barnard. I had the extreme pleasure recently of meeting him and sitting down to do an on-camera interview. He is the founder and President of the Physician's Committee for Responsible Medicine in Washington, D.C., which began in 1985. According to Dr. Barnard, "Our efforts are dramatically changing the way doctors treat chronic diseases such as diabetes, heart disease, obesity, and cancer. By putting prevention over pills, doctors are empowering their patients to take control of their own health, with plant-based diets." [32]

I found this piece of information, when I Googled people seeking answers to their health concerns, "Google receives more than one billion health questions every day. An estimated seven percent of Google's daily searches are health-related," according to Google Health Vice President David Feinberg, MD, *The Telegraph* reports. Google's total daily health-related searches amount to 70,000 each minute, according to the report.

Numerous doctors are at the tip of the spear for this whole food plant-based movement. Dr. Neal Barnard's book *Reversing Diabetes Without Drugs* saved my life. I got to meet him in person at the Plantrician Project's Annual International Plant-Based Nutrition Healthcare Conference in Oakland, California in September of 2019. It was an overwhelming experience to meet him, not only because he had such an impact on me but, also, because his work was so significant to my mother many years ago. I was honored that he took the time out of his busy schedule to meet with me to do a video interview. He was extremely gracious and informative.

Special Note: With each passing day we see the COVID-19 pandemic unfold.   Over and over, the deaths are predominantly those with "underlying conditions," particularly diabetes. Metformin is on the list of the Top 10 Most Widely Prescribed Drugs in the U.S. Because I have performed over 70,000 anesthetics over the past 32 years, I see what medications patients are taking. About 65% of my patients have diabetes, and they're all on Metformin. Right now, on the news, the drug for malaria is being touted as the miracle drug for COVID-19.   A study I just read is very frightening. Researchers warn that this malaria drug, hydroxychloroquine, may be toxic when combined with metformin. The research to date has been studied in rats, with deleterious results. This signals the need for "pharmacovigilance" when trialing on humans.[64]

My point here is that a vast majority of all individuals with Type 2 Diabetes can potentially decrease their metformin dosage and, in many cases, totally stop taking it by adopting the plant-based lifestyle, which has the potential of reversing their diabetes. The same holds true for heart disease, obesity, inflammatory diseases, and other conditions.

Chapter 28. The Tip of the Spear of the Plant-Based Movement

Neal Barnard, M.D. – Founder/President of the Physician's Committee for Responsible Medicine. Dr. Barnard's model for utilizing the whole food plant-based diet is my top choice for what other physicians should follow. To best hear it in his own words, please visit my website and listen to him discuss it at www.yourwfpblife.com

He encourages other physicians, residents, and medical students to come to the Barnard Medical Center to see first-hand how his system works. As he puts it, yes, he only has ten minutes or so with each patient, but he has a "whole Army" of staff who work with the patient to teach them what the whole food plant-based diet is, how to get started, how to cook for best effect, and all other things that are involved.

Obviously, a physician has very little time in just ten minutes to educate a patient about this lifesaving change. Nor can s/he simply tell a patient to go start a whole food plant-based diet and get up to walk out the door.

On his website, www.pcrm.org, you will find an extremely comprehensive source of information not only for physicians but for patients as well, from research results to recipes and everything in-between. PCRM offers free online continuing medical education for doctors, nurses, and dietitians to build their nutritional knowledge. Please visit https://www.pcrm.org/good-nutrition/nutrition-for-clinicians

They offer a free nutrition app for healthcare providers and extensive information for clinicians. On this page you will find what you need to help get started. The section with recipes is perfect for anyone starting the whole food plant-based diet. The recipes show the food and have easy-to-follow directions.[33]   It is a powerful site to find all the information you could possibly need to learn about the whole food plant-based diet, incorporate it into your practice, and direct all your patients to it as well.   It is a life-saving site, not just for diabetes but there's evidence it helps also with Alzheimer's, arthritis, breast cancer, cancer, colorectal cancer, diabetes, gut bacteria, healthy bones, heart disease, high blood pressure, migraines, prostate cancer, and weight loss.

In 2015, Dr. Barnard founded the Barnard Medical Center, which provides primary care and emphasizes diet and preventative medicine.   Dr. Barnard is a vegan. He has appeared on "The Dr. Oz Show" and "The Ellen Show." He's also a real-life rock star, with his band CarbonWorks! You can see more at www.carbonworksmusic.com [34]

T. Colin Campbell, PhD is one of the veterans of this movement, with his book *The China Study*. He was one of the lead scientists on diet and disease in the China-Cornell-Oxford Project, set up in 1983 by Cornell University, the University of Oxford, and the Chinese Academy of Preventive Medicine to explore the relationship between nutrition and cancer, heart, and metabolic diseases. The study was described by *The New York Times* as "the Grand Prix of epidemiology." This study appears to link the consumption of animal protein with the development of cancer and heart disease. He argues that casein, a protein found in milk from mammals, is "the most significant carcinogen we consume."[35] https://nutritionstudies.org/

Caldwell Esselstyn, M.D. – Another veteran of the whole food plant-based movement, he is the cardiovascular disease expert. Esselstyn is the author of *Prevent and Reverse Heart Disease* (2007), in which he argues for a low-fat, whole food plant-based diet that avoids all animal products and oils, as well as reducing or avoiding soybeans, nuts and avocados. Advocated by former U.S. President Bill Clinton and other famous people.[36] http://www.dresselstyn.com/

John McDougall, M.D. is the doctor who most vocally destroys the myths surrounding high carbohydrate diets. His message is that the main source of your calories should come from potatoes, rice, corn, and beans accompanied by vegetables and fruits. [37]

Dean Ornish, M.D. advocates using diet and lifestyle changes to treat and prevent heart disease. His work inspired and encouraged many of the other vegan doctors to pursue this path to treating patients by recommending a whole food vegan diet. Dr. Ornish is passionate about creating a healthy planet and healthy people by eating plant-based foods, exercising moderately, and including yoga and meditation in one's daily life. He allows for small portions of supplemental fish and oils and is not 100% vegan in his approach.[38] www.ornish.com

Michael Greger, M.D. – You can find the latest scientific findings about anything vegan and nutrition on Dr. Greger's website www.nutritionfacts.org He evaluates reputable studies to bring you the latest up-to-the-minute findings on a daily basis. His career was inspired by his grandmother. At the age of 65, she was literally sent home to die from her end-stage heart disease. She lived another 31 great years. thanks to Dr. Pritikin's program. Pritikin is one of the "lifestyle medicine" pioneers. Greger's grandma went from not being able to get out of her wheelchair to walking 10 miles a day from following Pritikin's advice. He became a vegan after touring a cattle stockyard early in his career. In 2005, "he joined the farm animal welfare division of the Humane Society as director of public health and animal agriculture. In 2008, he testified before Congress after the Humane Society released its undercover video of the Westland Meat Packing Company, which showed downer animals entering the meat supply, which led to the USDA forcing the recall of 143 million pounds of beef, some of which had been routed into the nation's school lunch program." [39]

Kim Williams, M.D. – Board certified in internal medicine, cardiovascular diseases, nuclear medicine, nuclear cardiology, cardiovascular computed tomography, he is now a professor and Chief of the Division of Cardiology at Rush University Medical Center in Chicago. He went plant-based the day he discovered his LDL cholesterol was 170 in 2003. A few weeks later, his LDL was within the normal range. He is quoted as saying, "there are two kinds of cardiologists: vegans and those who haven't read the data." He has a strong focus on the prevention of cardiovascular disease and encourages his patients to pursue the plant-based lifestyle.[40] https://www.plantbasednews.org/lifestyle/plant-based-cardiologist-dr-kim-williams-headline-nutrition-symposium-australia

Hana Kahleova, M.D., PhD., M.B.A. – Dr. Kahleova is the director of clinical research for the Physician's Committee for Responsible Medicine. She is an endocrinologist with a doctorate in human physiology and pathophysiology. Her current research interests include focus on dietary treatment of metabolic disease and Type 2 Diabetes. She conducted several clinical trials on the power of a plant-based diet to improve oxidative stress and metabolic control in patients with Type 2 Diabetes. www.pcrm.org 41

Laurie Marbas, M.D. – Dr. Marbas is double board certified in family medicine and lifestyle medicine. She has been following a whole food plant-based diet for the past five years in rural Colorado. At a large hospital in Colorado, she successfully created a lifestyle medicine program which is centred around the whole food plant-based diet. She speaks around the country at big conferences and is also the Managing Editor for the Plantrician Project's *International Journal of Disease Reversal and Prevention*.

Dr. Kim Williams is the Editor-in-Chief of the publication.[42] https://www.healthyhumanrevolution.com/store

Scott Stoll, M.D. – Dr. Stoll is the co-founder of the Plantrician Project, which has the Mission Statement, "To educate, equip and empower our physicians, healthcare practitioners and other health influencers with knowledge about the indisputable benefits of plant-based nutrition." [43]

Dr. Stoll is a highly sought-after international speaker and has appeared on numerous national shows including "The Dr. Oz Show" and numerous documentaries including "Eating You Alive," "Wait Till It's Free," and "The Game Changers." He is also an author and was a member of the 1994 Olympic Bobsled Team.[44] https://drscottstoll.com/

Hans Diehl, DrHsc, MPH, FACN – Dr. Diehl is the founder of the Lifestyle Medicine Institute in Loma Linda, California and the Complete Health Improvement Program (CHIP), a community-based education program educating physicians and patients alike about the power of nutrition as medicine. He is also Clinical Professor of Preventive Medicine at the School of Medicine of Loma Linda University. He has over 30 years in the emerging field of Lifestyle Medicine. [45] https://www.hansdiehl.com/

Michael Klaper, M.D. - Dr. Klaper has practiced medicine for more than 40 years and is a leading educator in applied plant-based nutrition and integrative medicine. He advocates plant-based diets and the end of animal cruelty. Dr. Klaper is now on another mission, to remedy the omission of nutrition education to medical students. Together with *PlantPure Communities*, his new *Moving Medicine Forward* initiative is "bringing the revolutionary ideas of disease reversal through plant-based nutrition and lifestyle medicine to medical schools across the country!" Visit Dr. Klaper's website https://www.doctorklaper.com/ to learn more. [46]

Garth Davis, M.D. – Dr. Davis is very active on social media with numerous outspoken TV appearances and is a very prominent vegan doctor. He is an Ironman Triathlete and a recovered "Proteinaholic," the name of his book. He specializes in bariatric weight loss surgery but is now recommending a whole food plant-based diet to his patients for best health and long-term weight loss/maintenance results. Dr. Davis gives talks all around the country on diet and its health implications and gives cooking classes, which he received training through the Physicians' Committee for Responsible Medicine's Food for Life Certification. He turned to the vegan diet at the age of 36 after discovering he had cholesterol deposits in his eyes during a routine exam. He also had hypertension, high cholesterol, and a fatty liver. Then he learned about the power of a plant-based diet. He now is also competing in marathons. He's featured in the famous documentary *What the Health*.[47] http://proteinaholic.com/

Joel Kahn, M.D. – PETA's 2016 "Sexiest Male Vegan Over 50!" is author of four books and a cardiologist. Dr. Kahn is a Professor of Medicine at Oakland University, William Beaumont School of Medicine, and manages his own Center for Longevity. He is also a columnist at *The Huffington Post* and *Readers Digest*. He believes that plant-based nutrition is the most powerful source of preventative medicine on the planet. He is also in in the documentary "What the Health." Having treated thousands of acute heart attacks during his career, he's educating people about the plant-based diet and holistic lifestyle to prevent ALL future heart attacks. On his ABOUT page, it states, "He passionately lectures throughout the country about the health benefits of a plant-based anti-aging diet, inspiring a new generation of thought leaders to think scientifically and critically about the body's ability to heal itself through proper nutrition." [48] https://www.drjoelkahn.com/

Susan Benigas and Tom Dunnam, MBA – Along with Dr. Scott Stoll, Susan and Tom are co-founders of The Plantrician Project and the International Plant Based Nutrition Healthcare Conference.   Susan has a passion for "reaching the gatekeepers of dietary recommendations—our nation's physicians and healthcare practitioners," which led to her founding The Plantrician Project and co-founding the International Plant-based Nutrition Healthcare Conference, showcasing the efficacy of whole food plant-based nutrition in its ability to prevent, suspend and often even reverse much of the chronic, degenerative disease afflicting our world." [49]

https://plantricianproject.org/

Chapter 29. Links and Suggested Reading for Physicians & All Healthcare Professionals

Physicians Committee for Responsible Medicine – pcrm.org

The Plantrician Project – plantricianproject.org

Documentaries:

- *The Game Changers*

- *What the Health*

- *What You Eat Matters*

- *Forks Over Knives*

- *Eating You Alive*

Books by Dr. Neal Barnard

Dr. Neal Barnard's Program for Reversing Diabetes: The Scientifically Proven System for Reversing Diabetes Without Drugs

Dr. Neal Barnard's *Cookbook for Reversing Diabetes: 150 Recipes Scientifically Proven to Reverse Diabetes Without Drugs*

Your Body in Balance: The New Science of Food, Hormones, and Health

The Vegan Starter Kit: Everything You Need to Know About Plant Based Eating

21-Day Weight Loss Kickstart: Boost Metabolism, Lower Cholesterol, and Dramatically Improve Your Health

The Cheese Trap: How Breaking a Surprising Addiction Will help You Lose Weight, Gain Energy and Get Healthy

Power Foods for the Brain: An effective 3-Step Plan to Protect Your Mind and Strengthen Your Memory

Foods That Fight Pain: Revolutionary New Strategies for Maximum Pain Relief

T. Colin Campbell, PhD

The China Study: Revised and Expanded Edition: The Most Comprehensive Study of Nutrition Ever Conducted and the Startling Implications for Diet, Weight Loss, and Long-Term Health

Whole: Re-Thinking the Science of Nutrition

The Low-Carb Fraud

The China Study Cookbook: Over 120 Whole Food Plant Based Recipes

The Campbell Plan: The Simple Way to Lose Weight and Reverse Illness, Using The China Study's Whole Food Plant Based Diet

The Plant Pure Kitchen: 130 Mouthwatering, Whole Food Recipes and Tips for a Plant Based Life

. . .

Caldwell Esselstyn, M.D.

Prevent and Reverse Heart Disease: The Revolutionary, Scientifically Proven, Nutrition Based Cure

The Prevent and Reverse Heart Disease Cookbook: Over 125 Delicious, Life-changing, Plant Based Recipes

Gene Stone

Forks Over Knives: The Plant Based Way to Health

Forks Over Knives- The Cookbook: Over 300 Recipes for Plant Based Eating All Through the Year

Rip Esselstyn

The Engine 2 Diet: The Texas Firefighter's 28 Day Save Your Life Plan that Lowers Cholesterol and Burns Away the Pounds

The Engine 2 Cookbook: More than 130 Lip-Smacking, Rib-Sticking, Body Slimming Recipes to Live Plant Strong

Plant Strong: Discover the World's Healthiest Diet with 150 Engine 2 Recipes

The Engine 2 Seven Day Rescue Diet: Eat Plants, Lose Weight, Save Your Health

Shushana Castle & Amy- Lee Goodman

Re-Think Food: 100+ Doctors Can't Be Wrong

Michael Greger, M.D.

How Not to Die: Discover the Foods Scientifically Proven to Prevent and Reverse Disease

The How Not to Die Cookbook: 100+ Recipes to Help Prevent and Reverse Disease

How Not to Diet: The Ground-breaking Science of Healthy, Permanent Weight Loss

John McDougall, M.D.

The Starch Solution: Eat the Foods You Love, Regain Your Health, and Lose the Weight for Good!

The McDougall Quick and Easy Cookbook: Over 300 Delicious Low-Fat Recipes You Can Prepare in 15 Minutes or Less

Scott Stoll, M.D.

Alive! A Physician's Biblical and Scientific Guide to Nutrition

Kristen's Healthy Kitchen Recipes

Dean Ornish, M.D.

Dr. Dean Ornish's Program for Reversing Heart Disease

Undo It! How Simple Lifestyle Changes Can Reverse Most Chronic Diseases

The Spectrum: A Scientifically Proven Program to Feel Better, Live Longer, Lose Weight, and Gain Health

Joel Fuhrman, M.D.

Fast Food Genocide: How Processed Food is Killing Us and What We Can Do About It

Garth Davis, M.D.

Proteinaholic: How Our Obsession with Meat is Killing Us and What We Can Do About It

Joel Kahn, M. D.

The Plant Based Solution

Vegan Sex: Dump Your Meds and Jump in Bed

Young at Heart by Design: A Program to Live Younger, Feel Younger, and Stay Younger

The No B.S. Diet

Dead Execs Don't Get Bonuses

Your Whole Heart Solution: What You Can Do to Prevent and Reverse Heart Disease Now

Kris Carr

Crazy Sexy Kitchen: 150 Plant-Empowered Recipes to Ignite a Mouthwatering Revolution

Jennifer McCann

Vegan Lunch Box: 130 Amazing, Animal-Free Lunches Kids and Grown-Ups Will Love!

Vegan Lunch Box Around the World: 125 Easy, International Lunches Kids and Grown-Ups Will Love

Dreena Burton

Plant-Powered Families: Over 100 Kid-Tested, Whole Foods Vegan Recipes

Let Them Eat Vegan! 200 Deliciously Satisfying Plant Powered Recipes for the Whole Family

Bryanna Clark Grogan

World Vegan Feast: 200 Fabulous Recipes from Over 50 Countries

A Food Revolution.

Now, there is a way to naturally address many of these diseases, which can be prevented, treated, and even reversed. Please take the time to do read, listen, and research all the information. Also, consider attending a plant-based healthcare conference to not only learn more about this revolution but connect with fellow physicians already using this in their everyday practice. You may also contact Dr. Neal Barnard to schedule a visit to the Barnard Medical Center to learn first-hand how to transition your medical practice to one which incorporates the plant-based lifestyle into the patient treatment model.

Part 4:
Meal Planning and Recipes

Chapter 30. How to Plan Your Plate and Recipes

Menu Planning

I want to give you a three-week look at ideas for your meals. One thing to remember is that you don't have to measure, weigh, count calories, or any annoying things like that. You can eat as much as you want, and you will never be hungry.

The foods you will be eating are rich in fiber and will fill you up and keep you full.

I personally don't have time on weekdays to prepare meals from recipes that involve numerous ingredients and steps. Those dishes are reserved for the weekend when I'm not pressed for time. I'm betting you know where I am coming from! What I do during the week is create hearty meals using the different things I cooked in bulk on Sunday. There is, of course, the option of making more complex meals and placing them into the freezer and take out as needed. Always be sure to put the date on everything, even if it is going in the freezer. Frozen foods are not good indefinitely. Three days is the maximum time I'll save anything in the refrigerator. I've read numerous sites that tell you things can last 3-5 days. I prefer to err on the safe side. I simply want to be sure to use up what I've purchased, so I don't have to feel bad about tossing the unused food into the trash. This might sound a bit funny, but I have an old-fashioned chalkboard in the kitchen that is used to keep track of food inventory, not only for food that got cooked but when food is brought home from the grocery store. I came up with this idea after totally forgetting I purchased the world's biggest artichokes, which ended up way back in the refrigerator.

Many days later, I was looking for something in the fridge and reached way in the back. I felt something squishy and nasty feeling. I slowly pulled the mystery bag out to discover those once-gorgeous artichokes were now beyond wilted, even leaking liquid! I had totally forgotten about them.

The solution was to write down all the different vegetables, fruits, and perishable items on the chalkboard. Then, you can keep track of what's on hand, not only to be sure you use them up, but you can quickly come up with recipe ideas by looking at the board. Plus, it's just cute to look at that board! I write it pretty using multiple colors of chalk. I love old-fashioned things, so the chalk board makes it cozy in the kitchen, the heart of the home.

You can now make your own chalkboard! There's special paint called "chalkboard paint," and you can put it on wood to make a board or use it to paint on cans or jars in which you can plant herbs. It allows you to write the name of the herb on the front of the can/jar with chalk, and it looks -- you guessed it -- old-fashioned! It's very simple to grow your own herbs at home, using empty containers as your garden! I use cilantro, basil, and parsley all the time, so, by growing my own, I never run out, not to mention they are simply a joy to look at.

Another tip regarding herbs. When you purchase them from the store, once home you can trim off the bottom of the bunch and place it into a glass of water and put it in your refrigerator. They will perk right up, look pretty, and are ready and fresh when you need them! Wash before using!

First, I want to go back and talk about the Power Plate that I mentioned earlier in the section under "Meal Planning." It has four sections – fruits, grains, legumes, and vegetables. Maybe print off that picture and put it up in your kitchen, so it's readily available to help guide you. Once you get the hang of it, meal planning and preparation will get easier. Below is a direct link to the PCRM site's section on the Power Plate specifically for diabetes.[50]

https://p.widencdn.net/4zgr4r/18301-DIA-Native-American-Recipe-Booklet-Update-final

Also visit https://p.widencdn.net/ktho8u/Power-Plate-Brochure [51] This is the main page for Power Plate information. There is a huge amount of resources, with great recipes, shopping lists, and all you need to get started to stick with the plant-based lifestyle. As you will soon learn, Dr. Neal Barnard and his extensive team leave no stone unturned! I still continue to use his website for information, up-to-date research findings,

Dr. Barnard's Blog, recipe ideas, and more. The site is continuously updated and expanded.

Following is what I eat, with some ideas to help you get started. I do not want to tell you to go only to the PCRM website. I would feel like I have abandoned you.

Breakfast Ideas

Oat Groats

I'm like so boring concerning breakfast! I eat my beloved oat groats and fruit just about every day, except maybe Saturday. So, what the heck is so great about oat groats? Typically, old-fashioned rolled oats are a great pick for breakfast, the kind that takes about 10-15 minutes to cook. Those are great too, but oat groats take it to a different level. You want to look for the kind that are organic *and* non-GMO because they are not just any oat groats,

First, I'll give you the bad news. Oat groats take longer to cook than rolled oats or steel-cut oats – up to an hour but typically 40-45 minutes. That's why I list them on the Sunday Bulk Cooking list. You can cook up a big batch in a big 6-8-quart Dutch oven or soup pot. Make enough for three days. Yes, that means Wednesday you'll need to cook up the next batch! It's easy to cook. For each measuring cup of oat groats, you add two cups water. So, for example, I am going to make four cups of oat groats, I place four cups of oat groats into the pot and add 8 cups of water. Bring it to a full boil; then turn down the heat to an "active" simmer and cover. Simmer for 45 minutes to an hour, stirring occasionally. Watch the pot closely, as the oats and water will want to boil up a few times! Simply mix it well, cover, and keep simmering. Remember to stir occasionally.

Once the water is all absorbed, shut off the stove and remove from heat. Use that time to chop other vegetables or get other things ready. Or, put on some soft, relaxing music, use some aroma therapy such as a simmering pot of cinnamon, nutmeg, cloves, and orange peel, and take this opportunity to calm your mind and body. Don't think of cooking as drudgery. Instead, look at it as a time to heal the mind, body, and spirit. Have you heard of mindfulness? Here's your big opportunity to begin practicing mindfulness! The World Health Organization (WHO) defines health as "a state of complete physical, mental, and social well-being and not merely the absence of disease or infirmity." [52] Like other whole grains, oat groats help fight Type 2 Diabetes and cardiovascular disease. They have great health benefits and also are high in fiber and mineral content. Each serving of oat groats, approximately 1 cup cooked, contains 150 calories, 6 grams of protein, 26 carbohydrates, and 4 grams of fiber. All of this helps maintain healthy tissue, a strong immune system, and fuel for your brain. The fiber helps lower your risk of cardiovascular disease and helps lower blood sugar. They contain iron and phosphorus, zinc, and copper.   There are many more nutrients. Altogether, this grain provides your body with a powerful symphony of nutrients to improve your health.

For breakfast, I like to add two to three different fruits as toppings: fresh blueberries, blackberries, raspberries, apples, bananas, mango, papaya, guava, kiwi, dragon fruit, cactus pear, pears, whatever you like. I vary the combination of fruits to spruce things up.   I also add a teaspoon of Ceylon cinnamon, one tablespoon freshly ground flaxseed and one tablespoon of ground hempseed, and, maybe, a tablespoon of chia seeds. You need to mix these dry items in before topping with fruit. If you desire, add some non-dairy unsweetened milk -- like unsweetened almond milk -- to thin down the oats to your desired choice of consistency.

Let me talk about apples for a moment.   Ever since my childhood, I have been eating an apple each day.   The only time I wasn't eating them was the nearly two years I was following that Keto diet.   When I started on the plant-based lifestyle, I was immediately back to eating one a day. So, over the past few months, I noticed that the several different kinds of apples I like seemed basically, tasteless: Honey Crisp, Fuji, and a new "breed," Cosmic Crisp.   I decided to write the company shown on the little sticker, about the one I started eating and discovered brown decay inside.   I cut it open to take photos to send them with my complaint. I received a call from the company with some fascinating news! The man explained that the brown "decay" I found inside that apple was actually fermentation caused by a process called "Controlled Atmosphere" storage. In CA storage rooms, the temperature, oxygen, carbon dioxide, and humidity levels are adjusted to form hospitable hibernation environments for apples being stored after harvest.

They are basically putting the apples to sleep. With a perfect combination of temperature and gases, which differs for each variety, it allows apples to stay fresh longer after harvest than if they were simply refrigerated. The lower the oxygen, the sleepier they can make the apples. Sleepier apples have slower respiration rates and stay firm, colorful, flavorful and nutritionally dense for longer. The trick is to avoid bringing the oxygen levels too low; otherwise, the apples ferment. So, basically, that apple in which I found the brown spots was an over-anesthetized apple! As an anesthesia provider for humans, I find this quite entertaining! Read more here: [53] https://www.npr.org/sections/thesalt/2018/11/26/668256349/thanks-to-science-you-can-eat-an-apple-every-day

You can also use cooked oat groats to add into a salad for a chewy texture or make an oat groats' salad with some chopped vegetables, greens, and your choice of dressing (one free of animal products and oil.) I mostly use freshly squeezed lime juice on my salads.

I have a recipe for several oil free dressings. For many more recipes for dressings, check out Dr. Barnard's books for reversing diabetes without drugs. Both the main book, *Dr. Neal Barnard's Program for Reversing Diabetes Without Drugs,* and his companion book, *Dr. Neal Barnard's Cookbook for Reversing Diabetes Without Drugs.* Between these two books, you will have several hundred great recipes for everything: breakfast, lunch, dinner, snacks, dressings, dips and more. These are all geared for individuals with diabetes and are scientifically proven to help reverse Type 2 Diabetes. You can find literally thousands of plant-based recipes on-line; however, even though they are plant-based, it does not guarantee they are diabetes friendly. You will learn to recognize this over time and learn what to substitute in order to make your recipe diabetes friendly!

Sorry for going off course: back to oats. Do feel free to use the old-fashioned rolled oats. They are perfectly fine. Just be sure you are not purchasing the instant oats. They are highly processed and worthless.

A further comment about oat groats. You will be pleasantly surprised how hearty they are and topped off with two or three different kinds of fruit, which makes it a special treat. Another point is about the cholesterol-lowering effect of oats. Research studies have determined that the more oats are processed, the less effective they are at lowering your cholesterol. Thus, oat groats are not processed at all, so they have the most potent ability to lower your cholesterol. That should put a smile on your face each morning as you fix your bowl of oat groats! I like to envision the oat groats going into my body and going through my veins like Ms. Pac-man, chomping away any residual cholesterol! OK, so who remembers Ms. Pac-man? [54] I have to admit to putting more than one quarter in the arcade machine to play that silly game! Here is another great breakfast idea, and it doesn't take too long.

Tofu Scramble

While there are a few prefabricated tofu scrambles available on the market, if you read the long list of ingredients, you are sure to find unwanted ingredients such as olive oil, too much salt, etc. So....it really isn't difficult to make this from scratch. It is so delicious, I suggest you make extra for dinner or use it as leftovers for the next day! You can store it up to three days in the fridge.

Ingredients
Spice Mixture
½ teaspoon Turmeric
½ teaspoon onion powder
½ teaspoon garlic powder
¼ teaspoon black pepper

2 tablespoons nutritional yeast

Salt: I suggest holding off on salt, as you can always add it to your food once it is cooked. That's my thoughts on salt for every recipe!

Tofu Scramble

1 12 oz. block of extra-firm tofu, crumbled

1 Red Bell pepper, chopped

1 small sweet onion, finely chopped

2 cloves garlic, minced

1 can Black Beans (2 cups), rinsed and drained

8 oz. mushrooms (white button or baby portobello), stems removed, sliced

1 cup (packed) greens of choice. I suggest baby Bok Choy, spinach, arugula

Vegetable broth (low sodium)

1. Place all the Spice Mixture ingredients into a small bowl and mix together. Set aside.
2. Heat a large non-stick skillet over medium-high heat. When hot, add the mushrooms, Red Bell peppers, and onions. Sauté for about 5-8 minutes, adding a dash of vegetable broth as needed to prevent sticking. This will be like adding 1-2 tablespoons at a time as needed. Do not add too much and make it soupy. You just want to add enough to prevent the mixture from sticking to the skillet. Continue sautéing until the

mushrooms/peppers/onions begin to brown/onions caramelize.

3. Add the tofu and mix well. Add the spice mixture and garlic, stirring well. Add the black beans, mixing well. Lastly, add the greens, mix well, and remove from heat.

4. Serve alone or with sliced tomatoes alongside, or vegetable of choice. I typically serve it with steamed broccoli on the side.

Sautéed Tofu

Occasionally I like to enjoy tofu for breakfast, sautéed in a skillet using low-sodium vegetable broth in place of oil or butter. I'll get a 12 oz. block of extra-firm tofu, place it on its side and cut it into about 5 one inch "slabs." I see some people call it tofu steaks, but I refuse to say that word. I call them tofu slabs or tofu pads.

Get the skillet hot, pour in a bit of the broth, add the tofu slabs and sauté until lightly browned, turning after several minutes. Add more broth as needed. These can be made in advance and stored in the refrigerator up to 3 days. They can be quickly heated and ready to eat in minutes.

You can make your meal by adding some vegetables of choice, some fruit, and a grain of some type.

You can also marinate the tofu slabs in a variety of diabetes/vegan friendly marinates. Get a big glass storage container. Place about a half cup of water, two tablespoons soy sauce, some freshly grated ginger, several cloves fresh garlic minced, and, maybe, some fresh turmeric root grated. Mix that all together, place the tofu slabs in it and refrigerate 30 minutes. Take out the container, turn each slab to marinate the other side, and return to the fridge another 30 minutes.

You can then either sauté these in a skillet or bake them for 30 minutes. I make up at least 10 slabs. In addition to meals, I place a slab wrapped in parchment paper and have it as my mid-morning snack. I might even take ¼ cup of black lentils to go with it or black rice.

Think outside the breakfast box!
You can be as boring as you'd like for breakfast or be daring and eat Bean Burritos for breakfast! There are no rules stating you must eat "breakfast" food for breakfast. The sky's the limit. Let's say you have a huge pot of vegetable soup in the fridge, and you're worried that it won't get used up within three days. Your options are either freeze it in separate containers or eat it for breakfast too!

Do try and eat greens several times a day. This is critical. Leafy green vegetables help maintain enough nitric oxide in your blood to help reduce your risk of cardiovascular disease. This topic in and of itself has endless books and research behind it. Feel free to Google it in your spare time.

Remember to rotate your greens, don't simply eat spinach leaves each day. Be adventuresome and try all the different greens you can find at the store. Remember to eat the greens from beets. They contain huge amounts of nutrients. Be sure to thoroughly wash these and any greens. If you can find beets with the greens still attached, you will see there's typically residual dirt on the leaves. Most people toss out those greens; unbeknownst to them, there are great nutritional value loaded in those greens.

Lunch and Dinner Ideas

One easy thing to keep on hand are sweet potatoes, orange or purple. I eat one a day, either at lunch or dinner. Or even as a snack. In my endless quest for knowledge, I discovered that sweet potatoes are a staple of the Okinawan diet and are eaten daily. You can prepare them either baked, roasted, steamed, or even made into soup.

Here is another idea: include **fermented foods** such as Sauer Kraut (the kind that must be refrigerated), miso paste (the kind that must be refrigerated), tempeh. These foods provide you with good bacteria to promote a healthy gut microbiome, the environment of bacteria that live in your gut, which potentially affects your immune system, your weight, and your risk for certain chronic diseases. Limit your consumption to small portions, however, as these foods do contain a lot of salt. I will eat a half cup of kraut or use some miso paste to make salad dressing. Fermented foods are important for those with diabetes[55]. https://www.wellthy.care/diabetes-diet-fermented-foods-benefits/

Salads are always an option. Dressings are fine to use as long as they are oil free and do not contain animal products. It is best to make your own dressing; then, you have full control of the ingredients. You will find a vast array of dressings in Dr. Barnard's books and on-line. Here's a few dressings that I made up.

Oil Free Green Goddess Dressing

1 cup unsweetened almond milk

6 teaspoons fresh lemon juice

1 ½ cups silken tofu (tightly packed)

1 teaspoon sea salt

1 tsp garlic powder

½ tsp onion powder

¼ tsp ground black pepper

1/8 tsp mustard powder

2 cloves garlic, peeled (I use 4 as I LOVE garlic!)

1 shallot, small/peeled

Fresh chives – I get the small plastic package in the produce area and use ½ of it

2 cups fresh organic parsley (just regular parsley, NOT Italian flat leaf) tightly packed

¼ cup plus 2 tsp white vinegar

Add all ingredients EXCEPT the white vinegar into a high-speed blender. Puree until smooth and creamy. Then add the white vinegar and puree for just a few moments until it is thoroughly blended.

Enjoy!

Miso Dressing

½ cup non-dairy unsweetened milk (almond or soy)

1 tablespoon white miso paste (only use the kind that needs to be refrigerated)

2 cloves garlic, peeled

2 pitted Medjool dates

Add all ingredients into a small blender or Ninja Bullet-type blender. Blend for about 45 seconds to one minute. This is very rich, so you don't need a lot. Refrigerate the unused portion for the next day.

Miso Vinegar Dressing

1 Tablespoon white miso paste

1 teaspoon Red wine vinegar

¼ teaspoon smoked paprika

1/2 cup unsweetened almond milk

Juice of 1 lime

Pinch of sea salt

Place all ingredients into blender and blitz for 30 seconds. This is exotic and can also be used on pasta as sauce.

Cilantro Avocado Dressing

1 cup cilantro (washed/rinsed/drained), packed

1 avocado, peeled/pitted

2 cloves garlic, peeled

½ cup non-dairy unsweetened milk such as almond or soy

1 large pitted Medjool date

Pinch of sea salt (optional, to taste)

Place all ingredients into blender and blitz 30 seconds.

Lunch and Dinner

I'm still doing pretty much what I started out doing when I went strict plant-based. Lunch and dinner are assembled depending on what I made up as the bulk foods.

Let's say I have these items:

Grains:

- Quinoa

- Winter Wheat Berries
- Barley
- Black Rice
- Spelt
- Bulgur
- Amaranth
- Corn (Polenta)

Legumes:
- Black Beans
- Black and Green Lentils
- Chickpeas (Garbanzo Beans)
- Split Peas
- Navy Beans
- Pinto Beans
- Tofu Slabs

I know I said you do not need to measure out your food, but I must use some frame of reference. Choose a grain and a legume, and start out with, say, half a cup of each on your plate. Let's say you picked out quinoa and a slab of tofu. Now add some greens, like baby kale, and a cut up tomato and half a cucumber sliced up. I also add a small sweet potato, either orange or purple, or some steamed broccoli. Add a fruit of your choice, and now your Power Plate is ready to go. Despite eating the same breakfast each day, I do like to vary my lunches and dinners to ensure I am getting the most nutrients.

You can also make this Power Plate into a Bowl, creating a salad. You can eat it hot or cold. Here's a recipe that I frequently make, only I swap out different grains and legumes, so there is never the same mixture every day. It is quick and easy, if you have those various foods cooked and ready to go.

Fun Lunch Bowl

½ cup quinoa

½ cup black rice

½ cup black beans (if using out of can, rinsed and drained)

½ cup chickpeas (as above if out of can!)

½ cup lentils (cooked)

½ cup Cannellini beans (same if canned, rinsed, and drained)

Half red onion, finely chopped/diced

½ cup corn (either frozen, or cut off the cob)

½ cup peas (frozen)

1 Red Bell pepper, seeded and chopped

1 Yellow Bell pepper, seeded and chopped

1 Green Bell pepper, seeded and chopped

1 Orange Bell pepper, seeded and chopped

1 cup firmly packed Cilantro, chopped

Optional: I recommend either mango or papaya, flesh cubed into bite sized pieces.

2 limes

Add all ingredients into large bowl except for limes. Gently toss until all mixed well. Now squeeze lime juice all over the food, gently tossing to be sure lime juice evenly distributed.

This will make up a huge bowl that can be used for two days. I add in something even more "entertaining," and that's wheatgrass. I chop up a big handful and top it on the salad. We grow our own. It is potent in nutrients, but some people may be allergic to it. I am not suggesting you eat it, simply stating what I do. If you are interested in wheatgrass, I highly suggest reading about it before consuming it. [56]

Of the numerous things I'm doing to get others on the plant-based lifestyle, I am teaching a class at a local health food store. Their Education Center has a full kitchen, and I do a presentation about the plant-based diet, talk about my success story, and give a cooking demonstration. I like to get all the attendees right up around the counter area to watch up close the food preparation. They also get to eat the food, which shows them how delicious food can be when cooked without oils or butters. It turns into a fun, social gathering, and everyone is going back for seconds and thirds! For the first event, I wanted to make something that would attract the locals. Since Mardi Gras was just around the corner, I decided to make New Orleans' Red Beans and Rice, without the andouille sausage, of course! The crowd was wowed, stating it was the best Red Beans and Rice they ever had! Coming from true southerners, that's quite a compliment! I did not, however, make the traditional white rice. I made Basmati rice, which has the lowest glycemic index of all white rice. Here's the recipe. For myself, I make the black rice. If you do make Basmati rice, choose Brown Basmati rice.

New Orleans Red Beans and Rice

Table Salt

2 pounds small red beans (about 4 cups) rinsed and checked for debris   Note: Camellia Brand red beans are best suited for this recipe, but not mandatory.

I medium yellow onion chopped fine (1 cup)

1 green Bell pepper – seeded and chopped fine (about ½ cup)

2 celery stalks – chopped fine (1/2 cup)

4 cloves garlic -peeled and minced (about 2 tablespoons)

1 teaspoon fresh thyme leaves

1 teaspoon smoked paprika

2 Bay leaves

½ teaspoon Cayenne pepper

½ teaspoon fresh ground black pepper

3 cups low sodium vegetable broth

6 cups water

2 teaspoons red wine vinegar, divided

2 tablespoons finely chopped fresh parsley

Brown Basmati rice – 4 cups cooked as you normally cook rice (I use a rice cooker – rule of thumb: however much rice you put into rice cooker, add water to be one inch above rice line)

Hot sauce of choice

To prep the beans, you have two options:

Overnight soak – Into four quarts of cold water, stir in two tablespoons salt and two pounds small red beans. Soak overnight at room temperature at least eight hours and up to 24 hours. Drain and rinse well.

Or

The "quick brine" method is great as well. I use this method. Using a large Dutch oven, place Four quarts water, two tablespoons salt, and two pounds small red beans. Bring to a boil over high heat. Remove the pot from the heat, cover, and let stand one hour. Drain and rinse the beans and proceed with the recipe. In a large Dutch oven over medium-high heat, let the pot get nice and hot (I put the timer on for two minutes). Add the onion, green pepper, and celery, stirring constantly. Continue stirring. The vegetables will start to stick to the bottom of the pot. Toss in 1-2 tablespoon(s) low-sodium vegetable broth and continue stirring.

Continue stirring and adding broth as needed to lightly brown the onions. They will begin to look caramelized, just as if you had used oil or butter. Once the onions are lightly browned and begin looking translucent, you are ready to proceed with the next step. Stir in garlic, thyme, paprika, Bay leaves, cayenne pepper, black pepper, cook until fragrant, about 30 seconds. Stir in vegetable broth, water, and beans and bring to a boil over high heat. Reduce heat and vigorously simmer, stirring occasionally, until beans are just soft, and liquid begins to thicken, about 45 to 60 minutes. Add one teaspoon red wine vinegar and stir well. Once the liquid has thickened, remove from heat, and add one teaspoon red wine vinegar and mix well again.

Ladle into bowls and top with a scoop of the Brown Basmati rice. Sprinkle the finely chopped parsley over the rice and beans. Serve with hot sauce of choice. Enjoy!
Another thing I regularly make, especially in the beginning of my plant-based lifestyle, is Dr. Neal Barnard's **Vegetarian Mixed-Bean Chili Express**. You can find this in his book *Dr. Neal Barnard's Program for Reversing Diabetes Without Drugs*, on page 232. It is delicious, and, as he says, it freezes well so you can put leftovers away. I have some Ezekiel bread with it and a side salad with lime juice or my Miso

Dressing on it.

Here's another one of my favorites, but this is from the companion cookbook, *Dr. Neal Barnard's Cookbook for Reversing Diabetes Without Drugs.* It's exotic and delicious! **Jamaican Stew**, on page 122. Make sure you squeeze the lime juice in it! I'm puckering up just thinking about it!

Gosh, I can't forget to mention the recipe for **Thai Corn and Sweet Potato Stew** on page 115.

I like exotic flavors which you will find in these and many more recipes. As I mentioned earlier, you can find thousands and thousands of plant-based recipes, but only the recipes found in Dr. Barnard's book are specifically for those with diabetes. Oh yes, I give you the recipes too for diabetes. Again, eventually you will learn what to exclude from any plant-based recipe and, instead, replace it with a diabetes-friendly version. For snacks, the list is endless. Here are some of the things that I'll make.

Corn Grits (Polenta) with Nutritional Yeast.

This is a great way to get your Vitamin B-12.

Stove Top:
-
- 1 cup Corn Grits/Polenta
- 3 cups Water
- 1/2 tsp Salt

Bring water and salt to a boil. Add Corn Grits and reduce heat. Cook slowly for about five minutes, stirring occasionally. Remove from heat, cover, and let stand for a couple minutes. This will make enough for four generous helpings. Add two rounded Tablespoons Nutritional Yeast to each serving and stir in. Enjoy!

Crispy Turmeric Roasted Chickpeas

2 cans Chickpeas, rinsed and drained and patted dry
1 teaspoon smoked paprika
½ teaspoon turmeric
1/8 teaspoon cayenne pepper
1/8 teaspoon ginger
Pinch sea salt

Pre-heat oven to 325 degrees F
Into large bowl add chickpeas and remaining ingredients. Toss to coat thoroughly. Pour onto cookie sheet lined with parchment paper. Bake 30 minutes. Turn oven off. Leave chickpeas in oven for 20 minutes. Remove from oven, set aside to cool. During cooling process chickpeas will get crispy. Serve as a snack, or in soups or salads.

Guacamole with Minced Garlic Dip and Red Cabbage Chips

I large ripe Avocado, pitted

2-4 cloves fresh garlic, peeled and minced

1/2 Fresh Lemon

Sea Salt

2 cups Red Cabbage cut into large pieces

Into bowl add avocado, minced garlic, juice of the lemon, and sea salt to taste. Mash the avocado and mix all ingredients well. Let sit for 15 minutes. This gives the enzymes in the garlic the time to form and provide the maximum health benefits.

Use the red cabbage "chips" to scoop up the guacamole!

Tempeh Mushroom Stroganoff

I just thought of this and want to share it. This is one of my favorite "treat" meals, usually for a Saturday evening dinner to eat by the fireplace.

2 pounds mushrooms (either portobello, shiitake or oyster)
   Stems maintained, thinly sliced

1 large sweet onion, peeled and diced

2 Packages Tempeh (8 oz. each) Original flavor, crumbled

1 carton vegetable broth low sodium

2 tablespoons white miso paste (the kind that is refrigerated)

2 cups unsweetened soy milk

2 large medjool dates, pitted

1 can Cannellini Beans, rinsed and drained

1 package frozen peas - cooked as directed on package

1 1 lb. package Ezekiel Sprouted Whole Grain Spaghetti

Boil spaghetti as directed on package. Drain and set aside.

Into Blender add the soy milk, dates, miso paste and Cannellini beans. Blend until smooth. Set sauce aside.

In a large non-stick skillet over medium-high heat, pre-heat skillet for two minutes. Then add the diced onion, and begin sautéing, stirring/mixing continuously. Add vegetable broth by the tablespoon as needed to prevent sticking. Continue sautéing until onions are lightly browned and fragrant. Add the mushrooms and continue to sauté until mushrooms lightly browned and tender. Add vegetable broth as needed, to keep from sticking or burning. Stir in the sauce followed by the tempeh and peas and lightly toss until tempeh and sauce are hot. Remove from heat. Quickly rinse spaghetti with hot tap water, drain thoroughly, then add to skillet. Gently fold pasta into the mixture. Serve immediately. Makes four servings. Top with freshly ground pepper and sea salt to taste.

Black Lentils with Nutritional Yeast

Combine ingredients in bowl: I cup cooked Black Lentils, heated to desired warmth and 2 Tablespoons Nutritional Yeast

Blueberries and Non-Dairy Yogurt

1/2 cup non-dairy unsweetened Almond Milk yogurt
   (I use Kite Hill Brand)
1/2 cup Blueberries (fresh or frozen)

Mix together in a bowl and enjoy!

A word about canned beans. If you are using canned chickpeas, save the fluid from the can. This starchy fluid is called "aquafaba," and it whips into a foam that can be used in baking and other ways. For great recipe ideas Google "aquafaba recipes" and visit www.beaninstitute.com

Chapter 31 – Boost Immune System Against COVID-19

I'm completing this book during the COVID-19 pandemic crisis. In fact, today's date is May 28, 2020. As of today, the numbers are as follows:

5.93 Million COVID-19 Cases Worldwide

358 Thousand Deaths Worldwide

United States now has over 100,000 Thousand deaths

Pre-existing Conditions:

> Cardiovascular Disease 13.2%
> Diabetes 9.2%
> Chronic Respiratory Disease 8.0%
> Hypertension 8.4%
> Cancer 7.6%

Also included are those who are immunocompromised and obese with a Body Mass Index greater than 40.

As I watch the crisis unfolding day by day, one factor is holding in place. Those with underlying medical conditions are faring the worst to this deadly virus, many of whom succumb despite ventilators and heroic efforts of medical personnel. Earlier, I talked about the global epidemic of heart disease, diabetes, obesity, hypertension, inflammatory diseases, and other common diseases. The World Health Organization is working towards reducing this world crisis of health conditions.

Now we have the Novel Coronavirus, COVID-19 raging a pandemic around the globe. I've already seen news segments about possible links to lifestyle habits, such as smoking and alcohol. I was holding my breath and sitting on the edge of my chair, waiting to hear them say "diet." Nope. Not a word. At least not from the media or public health researchers. But I see Dr. Barnard is right on top of it all, putting out interviews and videos linking food to health. What you put on your plate is the critical factor in your state of health.

At first, I thought this was the worst time to launch this book. As I began to see the death toll rise and hear over and over that it is linked to underlying health conditions, I realized that now is the EXACT time this book must be launched. I truly believe people around the world want to improve their health and build their immune system. Anyone can do it; you just have to want to do it to get your best health ever. There is no time better than right now.

The most important thing you can do to boost your immune system is eat the right foods. Although a strong immune system cannot occur overnight, now is the time to start giving your body the nutrients it needs to build strength. In addition to providing the immune boosting foods, you also need proper sleep, exercise, and stress-reduction to enable your body to function at full capacity.

The entire world is experiencing the devastating effects of the Coronavirus known as COVID-19. Globally, the death toll is rising every day. This lethal virus continues to spread. People are fearful not only of getting infected by COVID-19, but also of the evolving changes and restrictions of everyday life. It's difficult to keep from getting overwhelmed during this frankly, shocking time in history. This is exactly why you must not get so focused on the news that you forget to take care of yourself and your loved ones.

The CDC and World Health Organization are recommending safety measures such as frequent hand-washing, avoiding contact with individuals who are sick, avoiding events or areas where there are more than 10 people, avoid touching ,your face, practice good hygiene, wearing a mask, and self-quarantine for 14 days if exposed to a suspected case of COVID-19. And, of course, get tested if you develop any of the presenting symptoms, fever, sore throat, shortness of breath, or are exposed to an individual who is suspected/tests positive for COVID-19. In addition to all of this, you must build a strong immune system to help fight this deadly disease.

In very simple terms, your immune system is the group of cells and molecules that protect you from disease, bacteria and any foreign substance they perceive as threats. This includes COVID-19, a highly infectious microbe. Our immune system and gut flora (the healthy bacteria in our guts) work together with each other. The significance of their mutualistic relationship of supporting each other is in the fact that 70-80% of your body's immune system cells are located in your gut. [57]

In order for your immune system to function at its best, there must be a healthy interaction with your gut microbiota. Any kind of imbalance may alter your immune system responses. Therefore, gut health is critical, and it all starts with what you are eating. [58]

The bottom line is a healthy gut provides you with a strong immune system.

As I have already discussed earlier in this book, the foods that can cause inflammation in your body include animal products, sugar, high fructose corn syrup, processed meats, oils, refined carbohydrates, trans-fats, saturated fats, and artificial sweeteners. Remember I mentioned that artificial sweeteners negatively affect your gut flora? Also, dairy products cause inflammatory reactions in the small intestines and alter your immune system. [59]

When eating a whole food plant-based diet, you are getting a high intake of vitamins and low intake of fat, which helps have more effective white blood cells. It is the white blood cells that enable your immune system to produce antibodies to combat bacteria, viruses, and other invaders. Studies show that limiting dietary fat helps strengthen your immune defences. There are also many studies on oils which show that oil may impair your white blood cell functioning. Additionally, high-fat diets may alter that highly critical gut microbiota, thus compromising your immune system.[60]

Despite all of this, I haven't heard much of anything being said to eat foods that are known to boost the immune system during all the news coverage of COVID-19. Here and there will be a brief article, but not much more. As I mentioned earlier, though, a strong immune system is not built overnight. So, don't wait another second. Get started today.

Studies have shown that eating the right food and healthy lifestyle habits can boost your body's natural defense system. A whole food plant-based diet has been shown to give the immune system a boost. Foods that contain Vitamin C, Vitamin E, Vitamin A as beta-carotene, all help, as do foods rich in antioxidants which reduce oxidative stress. This diet will also decrease inflammation in the body.

Beta-carotene, for example, which is found in sweet potatoes, carrots, and green leafy vegetables, can reduce inflammation and boost immune function by increasing disease-fighting cells in your body.

Your immune system is also supported by Vitamins C and E, antioxidants that help to destroy free radicals. You can get Vitamin C from red peppers, broccoli, mangoes, oranges, strawberries, lemons, cantaloupe, kiwi, papaya, pineapple, raspberries, blueberries, cranberries, watermelon. Vitamin E is in nuts, seeds, broccoli, tomatoes, turnip greens, spinach, red sweet peppers, mango, kiwi.

Your white blood cells defend your body against invaders. Zinc is a mineral that can boost the WBC's, and you can get zinc from eating toasted wheat germ, firm tofu, hemp seeds, lentils, oatmeal, quinoa, shiitake mushrooms, black beans, green peas, spinach, white button mushrooms, lima beans, chia seeds, flax seeds, asparagus, pumpkin seeds, nuts.

I want to point out that instead of reaching for a bottle of supplements, there is no comparison to obtaining these critical nutrients from eating highly nutritious foods to obtain them. Nothing can beat Mother Nature's bounty!

I hate to say it, but it's really true, 'you are what you eat!' Make citrus fruits your best friends, as they contain high levels of Vitamin C which is critical for your immune functioning.

Green leafy vegetables are also highly important and remember to rotate your greens to get in a variety. Please do wash your greens in sudsy water. I fill a large bowl with cool water and a squirt of dish detergent. COVID-19 is an "enveloped" virus, meaning it is covered with an oily membrane. Because of this, soap is very effective at disrupting the oily surface and water is effective at removing and rinsing away the virus. Do not use vinegar washes as they are not known to be effective at killing viruses.

Get adventuresome with herbs, and experiment using them in your recipes. They are all excellent for your health, like oregano, thyme, garlic, basil, cilantro, parsley rosemary, ginger, and turmeric (root stalks).

Oh, yes, obesity. This is a global epidemic. It leads to diabetes, which is now why you may see the term diabesity. We keep seeing on the news that COVID-19 seems to be affecting those over 60 the most, who have underlying medical conditions like diabetes, heart disease, and obesity. You have the power to take control of what you eat, which in turn affects your health. As I state on the cover of this book, this *is A Food Revolution: How the Plant-Based Lifestyle Can Win the Global War on Diabetes, Obesity, and Heart Disease.* In addition, the plant-based lifestyle can help you build your immune system to its fullest capacity.

I also want to mention the seriousness of being overweight. Earlier in the book I shared with you of my weight problem that I struggled with my entire life. The plant-based way of eating immediately began melting the weight off. So far, I have lost

70 pounds, and I'm looking for another 50 to be gone. According to the World Health Organization, "In 2016, more than 1.9 billion adults aged 18 years and older were overweight. Overall, about 13% of the world's adult population (11% of men and 15% of women) were obese in 2016. The worldwide prevalence of obesity nearly tripled between 1975 and 2016."[61] I'm betting these numbers are far greater right now. There is strong research evidence that excess body weight has a negative impact on your immune functioning.[62]

I am not saying you will be immune to contracting COVID-19, or any other illness. I'm saying that you will have the best immune system you possibly can to help fight the insult, when you adopt the plant-based lifestyle. I'm scared. I'm sure you are scared. But I know that if I was at where I was 10 months ago before I started this, I know I wouldn't stand a chance of recovering, as my body was in a high state of inflammation, high blood pressure, high blood sugars, and 70 pounds heavier, chaos, all of which lowers the immune system.

Now is the time for a global paradigm shift of how people eat. Now is the time to go plant-based, not only for each person's best health possible, but for the positive impact it will have on our beautiful planet earth. This planet simply cannot sustain itself on the path it is on. There must be a dramatic change.

I recently received my Plant-Based Nutrition Certificate from the T. Colin Campbell on-line program from Cornell University. I highly recommend investing your time and money on this course. It is provocative, shocking, enlightening, and greatly informative. Dr. T. Colin Campbell, his son, Dr. Thomas Campbell, and other top experts, provide up to date information on the plant-based diet, as well the current state of our planet and the dire need to make this paradigm shift.

Plant-based protein can help end animal agriculture. Aside from the fact that eating plant-based is cruelty free, plant-based proteins do not contain the hormones or antibiotics found in factory-farmed meat. In a study at UCLA, "As for nutritional concerns: Pound-for-pound, gallon-for-gallon, animal-sourced foods use vastly more water and carbon to produce than plant-based foods. However; ounce-for-ounce, the amount of protein that you get from plant-sources, such as legumes, seeds, and grains, is closely on par, plus full of other healthful nutrients including fiber, sterols, stanols, and vitamins and minerals." [63]

To learn more about T. Colin Campbell Plant-Based Certificate,
https://www.ecornell.com/certificates/nutrition/plant-based-nutrition/

I use the word "boost" not to imply putting your immune system into "overdrive," but, instead, I mean to eat the right food to enable your immune system to function the way it is supposed to. When proper nutrients are not present, and harmful substances are instead ingested, your immune system cannot perform at its fullest capacity. Now, more than ever, we all need to jump on the plant-based movement to get your best health ever!

I would love to be part of your journey. Visit me at www.yourwfpblife.com

Chapter 32. Let Your Journey Begin

I know that life is all about choices. You have the choice of how you want your health to be. It might not seem easy at first, and you might encounter stumbling blocks. Don't worry about falling. Just be sure to get up and keep going. One of my favorite quotes is by Jon Bon Jovi, "Success is falling nine times and getting up ten."

Here's another one, by Henry Ford, "Obstacles are those frightful things you see when you take your eyes off your goal."

So, basically, what I'm saying to you is, even if you have a bad day and maybe don't stick to your plan as intended, don't give up. Get up, dust yourself off and get right back on track to reaching your goal. And remember to always ask yourself that *why* question. *Why* are you doing this? The answer remains the same. To get your best health ever, to feel good from the inside out.

Once you are plant-based for a while, not only will others notice your weight loss, but you will have that glowing look of "newly in-love!" When your body is functioning at its best capacity, inflammation is gone, and your health issues are under control or reversed, it shows on the outside. This is the best gift you could ever give yourself, which, in turn, is a gift to those you love, friends and family.

Hopefully, your success will inspire them to join you on your best journey ever!

Right now -- more than ever in history -- it is clear and important of to achieve your best health ever. While it is true that some individuals without any known health issues are succumbing to COVID-19, the vast majority do have one or more underlying conditions. Furthermore, there are countless people walking around with undiagnosed diabetes, heart disease, or some other condition.

Now is the time for that paradigm shift to the plant-based movement. YOU have the ability to take your health into your own hands. The time has come to begin your journey to your best health ever!

Cheers to you and your new PLANT-BASED Lifestyle!

I'd love to hear from you! Visit me at www.yourwfpblife.com

Special Thanks

I want to give **very special thanks to Dr. Neal Barnard for devoting his life's work to research on diabetes and his endless crusade of the plant-based movement.** I admire his tenacity of not being afraid to speak out about the meat industry, dairy and egg industry, and Big Pharma. Also, to applaud his tireless work for animal welfare.

I am extremely grateful to Dr. Barnard for taking the time out of his extremely busy schedule to sit down and allow me to interview him. His positive, gracious yet determined persona is infectious! He has had a very big influence on me since that encounter. I have applied what I learned from him to my journey of inspiring others to adopt the plant-based lifestyle.

My deepest thanks to my mom for teaching me how to cook and bake since I was a wee little girl, and for starting me out at an early age eating fresh fruits and vegetables throughout my entire life. I will never be able to forgive myself for not listening to my mom, when she wanted to go on Dr. Barnard's program back in 2006. I didn't have diabetes back then; nor did she. If we had, I would never have developed it, and I'm sure she would not have left this world when she did. The day I got to meet Dr. Barnard in person in Oakland, California was extremely overwhelming. First because he is so famous but also because that would have made my mom "over the moon." She planted the seeds in my mind of the plant-based diet, which enabled me to finally embrace it ten months ago. Yes, mom, Dr. Barnard is even more handsome in person than in photos!

I would also like to thank John Elbare, Director of Philanthropy, Southeastern Region, Physician's Committee for Responsible Medicine, for his help and ideas.

More thanks to Caroline Trapp, DNP, ANP-BC, CDE, DipACLM, FAANP, Director of Diabetes Education & Care, Physicians Committee for Responsible Medicine for her professional input.

I also want to thank Dr. Nguyen, the scheduling anesthesiologist, for eating that papaya which sparked a chain of events leading me to the plant-based lifestyle.

And of course, my **special thanks to Dr. Mimi,** for "entertaining" me with her presentation about the whole food plant-based diet, which prompted the door open in my brain, where I had the answers all along.

I also want to thank all the physicians listed in this book. They are all true pioneers, working tirelessly for what they believe in, because they know it's true from all the research-backed evidence. They are leading the crusade of the plant-based movement, which will enable individuals to achieve their best health possible. I stand to applaud them.

Last, but certainly not least, I want to **thank my husband Abraham,** for being there every step of the way. We are truly "The Team!" I love you, sweetheart, always and forever. And to our "Baby Cakes," there with me to help with yet another book. And our newest addition, Snowdrift, another rescue!

Author Bio

Anita Lesko is an award-winning author, national motivational speaker, and internationally recognized autism activist. She was a guest speaker at the **United Nations Headquarters** in New York City for World Autism Awareness Day 2017.

Anita received her Master of Science in Nurse Anesthesia from Columbia University in 1988, after which she embarked on her now 32-year career as a Certified Registered Nurse Anesthetist.

Anita is an Accredited Provider of AMA Category 1 Continuing Medical Education credits. She is also a Certified Life Coach.

After turning her life around with the plant-based lifestyle, Anita has turned her entire focus on helping others begin their journey towards achieving their best health possible. With the global pandemic of the COVID-19 crisis, Anita sees now as the time more than ever for people to immediately take charge of their health.

Anita would love to help you or your organization get started on a plant-based life! Connect with her at www.yourwfpblife.com

References

1. https://www.who.int/health-topics/diabetes
2. https://jamanetwork.com/journals/jamasurgery/fullarticle/400707
3. https://www.upmc.com/services/bariatrics/candidate/risks-and-complications
4. https://www.hsph.harvard.edu/news/press-releases/diabetes-cost-825-billion-a-year/
5. https://www.hsph.harvard.edu/news/hsph-in-the-news/worldwide-economic-burden-diabetes/
6. https://en.wikipedia.org/wiki/Hippocrates
7. Barnard, pg. xii, *Barnard, N. Reversing Diabetes Without Drugs*
8. Barnard, p. xv, *Barnard, N. Reversing Diabetes Without Drugs*
9. Barnard, p. xiv, *Barnard, N. Reversing Diabetes Without Drugs*
10. Barnard, N. *Reversing Diabetes Without Drugs*, pg. 25-28.
11. http://www.dresselstyn.com/site/why-does-the-diet-eliminate-oil-entirely/
12. https://www.youtube.com/watch?v=TYpnfr4jfTY
13. https://www.youtube.com/watch?v=iSpglxHTJVM
14. https://www.webmd.com/hypertension-high-blood-pressure/guide/grapefruit-juice-and-medication
15. https://www.healthline.com/nutrition/artificial-sweeteners-and-gut-bacteria#section3
16. https://www.youtube.com/watch?v=NlnOsnr94qM

17. https://www.youtube.com/watch?v=6ePOVdppS5s

18. https://www.mamasezz.com/

19. https://www.washingtonian.com/2014/03/25/food-diaries-how-george-washington-universitys-dr-neal-barnard-eats-for-a-day/

20. https://www.youtube.com/watch?v=kjZUQb19fWg

21. https://en.wikipedia.org/wiki/KISS_principle

22. https://www.businessinsider.com/annual-food-poisoning-deaths-2015-12

23. https://www.healthline.com/nutrition/foods-that-cause-food-poisoning#section4

24. https://www.healthline.com/nutrition/foods-that-cause-food-poisoning#section8

25. https://www.healthline.com/nutrition/foods-that-cause-food-poisoning#section9

26. https://jamanetwork.com/journals/jamanetworkopen/fullarticle/2758742

27. https://fungi.com/blogs/articles/place-mushrooms-in-sunlight-to-get-your-vitamin-d

28. https://pcrm1.ultracartstore.com/shop/literature/single/Kit-104.html

29. https://chironhealth.com/telemedicine/what-is-telemedicine/

30. https://www.mindbodygreen.com/0-8646/the-dangers-of-dairy.html
31. https://www.youtube.com/watch?v=Jf44vLndiRM

32. https://www.pcrm.org/about-us
33. https://www.pcrm.org/good-nutrition/plant-based-diets/recipes
34. www.carbonworksmusic.com
35. https://en.wikipedia.org/wiki/T._Colin_Campbell
36. https://en.wikipedia.org/wiki/Caldwell_Esselstyn

37. https://nutriciously.com/vegan-doctors/

38. https://nutriciously.com/vegan-doctors/

39. https://en.wikipedia.org/wiki/Michael_Greger

40. https://doctors.rush.edu/details/1728/kim-williams-sr-cardiovascular_disease-chicago-oak_park

41. https://www.pcrm.org/about-us/staff/hana-kahleova

42. https://www.healthyhumanrevolution.com/store

43. https://plantricianproject.org/vision

44. https://drscottstoll.com/
45. https://www.truehealthinitiative.org/council_member/hans-diehl/
46. https://www.doctorklaper.com/

47. http://proteinaholic.com/

48. https://www.drjoelkahn.com/

49. https://plantricianproject.org/board-of-directors
50. https://p.widencdn.net/4zgr4r/18301-DIA-Native-American-Recipe-Booklet-Update-final
51. https://www.pcrm.org/search?keys=power+plate
52. https://www.who.int/about/who-we-are/constitution
53. https://www.npr.org/sections/thesalt/2018/11/26/668256349/thanks-to-science-you-can-eat-an-apple-every-day
54. https://www.ncbi.nlm.nih.gov/pmc/articles/PMC5885279/
55. https://www.wellthy.care/diabetes-diet-fermented-foods-benefits/
56. https://www.healthline.com/health/food-nutrition/wheatgrass-benefits
57. https://neurohacker.com/how-the-gut-microbiota-influences-our-immune-system
58. https://neurohacker.com/how-the-gut-microbiota-influences-our-immune-system
59. https://darouwellness.com/dairy-one-of-the-biggest-immune-system-stressors/
60. https://www.pcrm.org/news/blog/foods-boost-immune-system
61. https://www.who.int/news-room/fact-sheets/detail/obesity-and-overweight
62. https://www.ncbi.nlm.nih.gov/pubmed/22414338
63. https://www.sustain.ucla.edu/our-initiatives/food-systems/the-case-for-plant-based/
64. https://www.who.int/docs/default-source/coronavirus/who-china-joint-mission-on-covid-19-final-report.pdf

65. https://www.who.int/docs/default-source/coronaviruse/who-china-joint-mission-on-covid-19-final-report.pdf

66. https://www.forbes.com/sites/victoriaforster/2020/04/05/researchers-warn-that-covid-19-treatment-touted-by-trump-may-be-toxic-when-combined-with-diabetes-drug/#77c7bd4255f8

.

Made in United States
North Haven, CT
27 May 2022

19601814R00136